101 BIBLE
Short Stories

Short Stories for Seniors

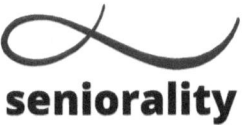

101 Bible Short Stories -
Jamie Stonebridge, Adam Harpwood
Copyright © 2024
Seniorality / Everbreeze Media Oy
Set in 16 pt EB Garamond

1. The Creation of the World

Genesis 1:1-31

In the beginning, God created the heavens and the earth. The earth was formless and empty, and darkness covered the deep waters. Then God said, "Let there be light," and there was light. God saw that the light was good, so he separated the light from the darkness. He called the light "day" and the darkness "night."

On the second day, God created the sky above and separated the waters below from the waters above. He called the sky "sky."

On the third day, God gathered the waters together, revealing dry ground. He called the dry ground "land" and the gathered waters "seas." Then God made plants and trees grow on the land, each bearing seed according to its kind.

On the fourth day, God created the sun, moon, and stars to light up the earth and to govern the day and night.

On the fifth day, God filled the seas with fish and the sky with birds. He blessed them, saying, "Be fruitful and multiply."

On the sixth day, God made land animals, each according to its kind. Then God said, "Let us make human beings in our image, to be like us." So God created human beings in his own image. He blessed them and told them to be fruitful and multiply, to fill the earth and govern it.

On the seventh day, God rested from all his work. He blessed the seventh day and set it apart as a special day of rest.

And so, God finished his creation, declaring it to be very good.

2. Adam and Eve in the Garden of Eden

Genesis 2:8-25; Genesis 3:1-24

In the beginning, God created a beautiful garden called Eden. He placed Adam, the first man, in the garden and gave him the job of taking care of it. God saw that Adam needed a companion, so He created Eve, the first woman, from one of Adam's ribs.

Adam and Eve lived happily in Eden, surrounded by lush trees, flowing rivers, and abundant fruits. They enjoyed the company of each other and walked with God in the cool of the day.

In the midst of the garden stood two special trees: the tree of life and the tree of the knowledge of good and evil. God warned Adam and Eve not to eat from the tree of the knowledge of good and evil, for if they did, they would surely die.

One day, a cunning serpent approached Eve and deceived her into eating the forbidden fruit. Eve, in turn, offered the fruit to Adam, and he also ate it.

Their eyes were opened, and they realized they were naked. Feeling ashamed, they sewed fig leaves together to cover themselves. When they heard God walking in the garden, they hid from Him.

God called out to them, and they confessed their disobedience. As a consequence of their actions, God cursed the serpent, Eve, and Adam. He banished them from the garden of Eden, where they had once known only peace and harmony.

Adam and Eve's disobedience introduced sin into the world, leading to pain, suffering, and separation from God. Yet, even in their disobedience, God showed mercy by promising a Savior who would one day redeem humanity from sin and restore fellowship with God.

3. Cain and Abel

Reference: Genesis 4:1-16

Adam and Eve, the first humans, had two sons named Cain and Abel. Cain worked the land, growing crops, while Abel tended to the flocks of sheep.

When the time came to offer sacrifices to God, Abel brought the best of his flock as an offering to God, showing his respect and devotion. Cain also offered a sacrifice, but it was not from the best of his crops.

God was pleased with Abel's offering, but He did not accept Cain's. This made Cain very angry and jealous of his brother.

One day, while they were in the field, Cain lured Abel into an argument and then killed him out of jealousy. When God asked Cain where Abel was, Cain lied, saying he didn't know.

But God knew the truth. He confronted Cain and pronounced a curse upon him. From then on, Cain would be a restless wanderer on the earth.

Feeling the weight of his guilt and the severity of his punishment, Cain lamented his fate. He feared that others would seek vengeance against him for what he had done.

In His mercy, God placed a mark on Cain to protect him from anyone who might harm him. Despite Cain's terrible deed, God still showed him mercy and gave him a chance to live.

Cain left the presence of God and went to live in the land of Nod, east of Eden, where he began a life of wandering and solitude, forever marked by the consequences of his jealousy and sin.

The story of Cain and Abel serves as a cautionary tale about the dangers of jealousy and the consequences of giving in to sinful desires. It reminds us of the importance of controlling our emotions and treating others with kindness and respect.

4. Noah's Ark

Reference: Genesis 6:9-22; Genesis 7:1-24 Genesis 8:1-22; Genesis 9:1-17

Long ago, in a time when the world was filled with wickedness, there was a man named Noah. Noah was a good man, and God saw that he was righteous among all the people.

God spoke to Noah and told him about a great flood that would cover the earth, wiping away all living things. But God promised to save Noah and his family if he built an ark—a huge boat—to keep them safe.

Noah obeyed God's command without question. He gathered wood and built the ark just as God instructed. It was a massive boat with many rooms and compartments.

Then, God told Noah to gather pairs of every kind of animal—male and female—to bring them onto the ark. Noah did as God asked, and the animals came to him, from the smallest ants to the biggest elephants.

When everything was ready, the rain began to fall. It poured down from the sky for forty days and forty nights, covering the earth in water. But Noah and his family were safe inside the ark.

For many days, the rain continued, and the waters rose higher and higher, until even the tallest mountains were covered. But the ark floated on the surface, keeping Noah, his family, and all the animals safe.

Finally, after many months, the rain stopped, and the floodwaters began to recede. The ark came to rest on the top of a mountain.

Noah waited patiently for the waters to go down. When the land was dry again, God told Noah it was time to leave the ark. Noah and his family, along with all the animals, stepped out onto the dry ground, grateful for God's protection and promise never to flood the earth again.

And in the sky, God placed a rainbow as a sign of His covenant—a promise of peace and protection for all generations to come.

5. The Tower of Babel

Genesis 11:1-9

In the land of Shinar, the people decided to build a great city with a tower that reached up to the heavens. They wanted to make a name for themselves and avoid being scattered across the earth.

The people worked hard, making bricks and using tar for mortar. They built the tower, layer upon layer, reaching higher and higher into the sky.

But God looked down from heaven and saw what the people were doing. He knew their intentions and saw that their pride and arrogance were leading them away from Him.

To humble the people and prevent their prideful ambitions, God decided to confuse their language. Suddenly, the people could no longer understand each other's words. They spoke in different languages, causing confusion and chaos.

Unable to communicate effectively, the people abandoned their construction project and scattered across the earth, each group speaking their own language and going their separate ways.

The tower, which came to be known as the Tower of Babel, remained unfinished, a reminder of the consequences of human pride and disobedience.

Through the story of the Tower of Babel, God demonstrated His sovereignty over humanity and His desire for people to trust and obey Him rather than relying solely on their own strength and ambitions.

6. Abraham's Call

Genesis 12:1-9

In the land of Ur, there lived a man named Abram, later known as Abraham. One day, God spoke to Abram, saying, "Leave your country, your family, and your father's house, and go to the land that I will show you."

God promised to bless Abram and make him into a great nation. He assured Abram that he would be a blessing to others, and all the families of the earth would be blessed through him.

Without hesitation, Abram obeyed God's command. He gathered his wife Sarai, his nephew Lot, and all their possessions, and set out for the land of Canaan.

As Abram journeyed through the land, God appeared to him and said, "To your offspring, I will give this land." Abram built an altar there and worshiped the Lord, grateful for God's promise.

Abram continued his journey, traveling from place to place, always following God's guidance. Along the way, he encountered challenges and trials, but he remained faithful to God's call.

Abram's faith and obedience pleased God, and He reaffirmed His covenant with Abram, promising to make his descendants as numerous as the stars in the sky and the sand on the seashore.

Through Abram's call, God demonstrated His faithfulness and sovereignty. He chose Abram and his descendants to be a light to the nations, fulfilling His plan to bring salvation to all people through the promised Messiah, Jesus Christ.

7. Abraham and Sarah's Journey

Genesis 12:10-20; Genesis 20:1-18

Abraham and Sarah embarked on a journey of faith, trusting in God's promises despite the challenges they faced.

As they traveled to the land of Canaan, they encountered a severe famine. Fearful for their well-being, Abraham decided to go to Egypt, believing they would find food there.

But as they approached Egypt, Abraham became anxious about Sarah's beauty. He feared that the Egyptians would kill him to take her as their own. So, he devised a plan, asking Sarah to say she was his sister, not his wife.

Sure enough, when they entered Egypt, the Egyptians noticed Sarah's beauty and praised her to Pharaoh. Thinking she was Abraham's sister, Pharaoh took her into his palace, and Abraham received many gifts because of her.

However, God intervened to protect Sarah and Abraham. He sent plagues upon Pharaoh's household, and Pharaoh realized the truth—that Sarah was Abraham's wife, not his sister.

Pharaoh confronted Abraham and questioned why he had deceived him. He then commanded Abraham and Sarah to leave Egypt immediately.

Despite this setback, Abraham and Sarah continued their journey, returning to the land of Canaan. Along the way, they faced other challenges, including conflicts with neighboring kings and the longing for a child.

Later in their journey, when Abraham and Sarah settled in Gerar, Abraham again feared for his life because of Sarah's beauty. He asked her to say she was his sister once more, leading to a similar situation with King Abimelech.

But once again, God intervened to protect Sarah and Abraham. He warned Abimelech in a dream not to touch Sarah, for she was Abraham's wife. Abimelech returned Sarah to Abraham and gave them gifts, acknowledging God's favor upon them.

Through their journey, Abraham and Sarah learned to trust in God's faithfulness, even in times of uncertainty and fear. Despite their shortcomings and mistakes, God remained faithful to His promises, guiding them on their journey and fulfilling His plan for their lives.

8. Abraham's Sacrifice of Isaac

Genesis 22:1-19

Abraham's faith was put to the ultimate test when God asked him to sacrifice his beloved son, Isaac.

One day, God called out to Abraham, saying, "Take your son, your only son Isaac, whom you love, and go to the land of Moriah. Offer him there as a burnt offering on one of the mountains of which I shall tell you."

Abraham, though deeply troubled, obeyed God without question. Early the next morning, he took Isaac and set out for the place God had shown him.

As they journeyed, Isaac asked his father, "Where is the lamb for the burnt offering?" Abraham replied, "God will provide the lamb, my son."

When they reached the designated place, Abraham built an altar and arranged the wood. Then he bound Isaac and placed him on the altar, ready to sacrifice him.

Just as Abraham raised his knife to slay his son, the angel of the Lord called out to him from heaven, saying, "Abraham, Abraham, do not lay your hand on the boy or do anything to him, for now I know that you fear God, seeing you have not withheld your son, your only son, from me."

Abraham looked up and saw a ram caught in a thicket by its horns. He took the ram and offered it as a burnt offering in place of his son.

God was pleased with Abraham's faithfulness and provided a ram as a sacrifice. He reaffirmed His covenant with Abraham, promising to bless him abundantly and make his descendants as numerous as the stars in the sky and the sand on the seashore.

Through Abraham's willingness to sacrifice his son, God foreshadowed the ultimate sacrifice of His own Son, Jesus Christ, who would one day die for the sins of humanity. Abraham's act of faith serves as a powerful testament to the obedience and trust we should have in God, even when His commands seem difficult to understand.

9. Jacob's Ladder

Genesis 28:10-22

Jacob, the son of Isaac and grandson of Abraham, embarked on a journey to find a wife from his mother's family. As night fell, he stopped to rest in a certain place, using a stone for a pillow.

While Jacob slept, he had a remarkable dream. He saw a ladder stretching from earth to heaven, with angels ascending and descending upon it. At the top of the ladder stood the Lord God.

God spoke to Jacob in the dream, saying, "I am the Lord, the God of your father Abraham and the God of Isaac. I will give you and your descendants the land on which you are lying. Your descendants will be as numerous as the dust of the earth, and through them, all the families of the earth will be blessed. I am with you and will watch over you wherever you go. I will not leave you until I have done everything I have promised you."

When Jacob awoke from his sleep, he was filled with awe and said, "Surely the Lord is in this place, and I was not aware of it." He took the stone he had used as a pillow and set it up as a pillar, pouring oil on top of it as an offering to God.

Jacob named the place Bethel, meaning "house of God," and vowed, "If God will be with me and watch over me on this journey, and if He will give me food to eat and clothes to wear so that I return safely to my father's household, then the Lord will be my God, and this stone that I have set up as a pillar will be God's house."

Filled with gratitude and reverence, Jacob continued his journey, knowing that the Lord was with him, guiding and protecting him every step of the way.

10. Jacob and Esau's Rivalry

Genesis 25:19-34; Genesis 27:1-46
Genesis 32:22-32

Jacob and Esau were twin brothers, born to Isaac and Rebekah. From the moment they were conceived, they struggled against each other in their mother's womb, foreshadowing the rivalry that would define their relationship.

Esau, the firstborn, was a skilled hunter and favored by his father Isaac. Jacob, on the other hand, was a quiet and cunning man, favored by his mother Rebekah.

Their rivalry became apparent when Esau, exhausted from hunting, returned home famished. Jacob, seizing the opportunity, offered Esau a bowl of stew in exchange for his birthright—the privilege and inheritance of the firstborn.

Esau, driven by his immediate hunger, foolishly agreed and sold his birthright to Jacob. This act of deception deepened the animosity between the brothers.

As Isaac grew old and his eyesight failed, he desired to bless Esau, his favorite son, before his death. Rebekah, overhearing Isaac's intentions, devised a plan to secure the blessing for Jacob instead.

Disguised as Esau with the help of animal skins, Jacob approached his father and received the blessing meant for his brother. When Esau learned of this deception, he was filled with rage and vowed to kill Jacob.

Fearing for his life, Jacob fled from his home and sought refuge with his uncle Laban. Over the years, Jacob prospered and grew wealthy while serving Laban, but he remained estranged from Esau.

Eventually, Jacob decided to return to his homeland, fearing Esau's wrath. On the night before their reunion, Jacob wrestled with a mysterious man, whom some believe to be an angel of God. Despite sustaining an injury, Jacob persevered and received a blessing, along with a new name—Israel, which means "he struggles with God."

When Jacob finally met Esau, he was surprised to find his brother forgiving and welcoming. Their reconciliation marked the end of their bitter rivalry and the beginning of a new chapter in their relationship.

11. Joseph's Coat of Many Colors

Genesis 37:1-11

Joseph, the son of Jacob, was favored by his father above all his brothers. To show his love for Joseph, Jacob made him a coat of many colors, a garment of rich and vibrant hues.

Joseph's brothers grew jealous and resentful of him because of their father's favoritism. To make matters worse, Joseph had dreams in which he saw himself as a ruler, and his brothers bowing down to him.

One day, Joseph shared his dreams with his brothers, unaware of the anger and envy they would provoke. His brothers scorned him and plotted against him, seeking to rid themselves of the object of their jealousy.

When Jacob sent Joseph to check on his brothers as they tended to their flocks, they saw an opportunity to get rid of him. They conspired to kill him and throw him into a pit, intending to deceive their father into believing he had been killed by a wild animal.

But Reuben, the eldest brother, intervened and persuaded the others not to shed Joseph's blood. Instead, they stripped him of his coat of many colors and threw him into a pit.

Later, as they sat down to eat, they saw a caravan of Ishmaelite traders passing by. Judah, another brother, proposed selling Joseph to the traders instead of killing him.

The brothers agreed, and Joseph was sold into slavery for twenty pieces of silver. They dipped Joseph's coat in goat's blood and presented it to their father, leading Jacob to believe that Joseph had been killed by a wild animal.

Meanwhile, Joseph was taken to Egypt, where he would face many trials and tribulations. Little did he know that his colorful coat would become a symbol of his father's love and his brothers' jealousy, setting in motion a chain of events that would ultimately lead to his rise to power and reconciliation with his family.

12. Joseph Sold into Slavery

Genesis 37:12-36

Joseph, the beloved son of Jacob, set out to check on his brothers who were tending to their father's flocks. As he approached them, they saw him from a distance and conspired against him due to their jealousy.

"Here comes that dreamer!" they said to one another. "Let's kill him and throw him into one of these pits. Then we'll see what becomes of his dreams."

But Reuben, the eldest brother, intervened, saying, "Let's not take his life. Instead, let's throw him into this pit in the wilderness, but don't lay a hand on him."

Reuben planned to rescue Joseph later and return him to his father.

So, when Joseph came to his brothers, they stripped him of his ornate robe, the coat of many colors, and threw him into an empty cistern.

As they sat down to eat, they saw a caravan of Ishmaelite traders approaching. Judah, another brother, suggested selling Joseph to the traders instead of leaving him to die in the pit.

The brothers agreed, and they pulled Joseph out of the pit and sold him to the Ishmaelites for twenty shekels of silver. The traders then took Joseph to Egypt.

When Reuben returned to the pit and found it empty, he tore his clothes in distress. The brothers took Joseph's robe, dipped it in goat's blood, and brought it to their father Jacob, saying, "We found this. Examine it to see whether it is your son's robe."

Jacob recognized the robe and concluded that a wild animal had killed Joseph. He mourned for his son in deep distress, refusing to be comforted.

Meanwhile, Joseph was taken to Egypt, where he would face many trials and hardships. Little did he know that God had a plan for him, even in the midst of his suffering, and that his journey would ultimately lead to great blessings and redemption.

13. Joseph Interprets Pharaoh's Dreams

Genesis 41:1-36

In the land of Egypt, Pharaoh, the ruler of the land, had troubling dreams that left him anxious and troubled. In his dreams, Pharaoh saw seven healthy and well-fed cows grazing by the Nile River, followed by seven thin and sickly cows that devoured the healthy ones. He also dreamed of seven plump and good ears of corn growing on one stalk, followed by seven thin and withered ears that swallowed up the healthy ones.

Disturbed by the dreams' meaning, Pharaoh called upon his wise men and magicians to interpret them, but none could provide an explanation that satisfied him.

At that time, Joseph, who was once a Hebrew slave but had risen to a position of authority in Egypt, was remembered by Pharaoh's cupbearer. He recounted how Joseph had interpreted his dream while they were both in prison.

Upon hearing this, Pharaoh summoned Joseph from the prison and told him his dreams.

Joseph listened carefully and then spoke under the guidance of God's wisdom, saying, "Both dreams have the same meaning. They signify that there will be seven years of abundance in the land of Egypt, followed by seven years of famine. The seven good cows and the seven good ears represent the years of plenty, and the seven thin cows and the seven withered ears represent the years of famine."

Joseph continued, advising Pharaoh to appoint a wise and discerning man to oversee the land during the years of plenty, storing up grain in preparation for the coming famine.

Impressed by Joseph's interpretation and wisdom, Pharaoh recognized the hand of God upon him and appointed him as the ruler over all of Egypt, second only to Pharaoh himself.

Thus, Joseph's God-given ability to interpret dreams not only saved Egypt from the impending famine but also elevated him to a position of great influence and power, fulfilling the purpose God had for him in the land of Egypt.

14. Joseph Reunited with His Brothers

Genesis 45:1-15

After Joseph's rise to power in Egypt, a severe famine struck the land, affecting many nations, including Joseph's family back in Canaan.

Jacob, Joseph's father, sent his sons to Egypt to buy grain, unaware that Joseph was alive and ruling in Egypt.

When Joseph's brothers arrived in Egypt and bowed before him, Joseph recognized them immediately. However, he disguised himself and spoke harshly to them, accusing them of being spies.

The brothers explained that they were honest men, sons of one man back in Canaan, and that they had come to buy grain to feed their starving family.

Joseph continued to test them, detaining Simeon as a hostage and instructing the others to return to Canaan and bring back their youngest brother, Benjamin, to prove their honesty.

Filled with guilt and fear, the brothers returned home and told Jacob everything that had happened. Jacob was distraught at the thought of losing another son and refused to let Benjamin go.

But as the famine persisted and their grain supply dwindled, Jacob had no choice but to send his sons back to Egypt with Benjamin, along with double the money they had paid for the grain and gifts for the Egyptian ruler.

When Joseph saw Benjamin with his brothers, he was overcome with emotion. He ordered his servants to prepare a meal and invited his brothers to dine with him.

Unable to contain his emotions any longer, Joseph revealed his true identity to his brothers, saying, "I am Joseph, your brother, whom you sold into slavery. But do not be distressed or angry with yourselves because you sold me here, for God sent me before you to preserve life."

Joseph embraced his brothers and wept openly, forgiving them for their past actions and expressing gratitude for God's providence in their lives.

Filled with joy and relief, Joseph's brothers embraced him in return, realizing that their reunion was a result of God's mercy and forgiveness. Together, they celebrated their newfound reconciliation and the restoration of their family.

15. Moses in the Bulrushes

Exodus 2:1-10

In the land of Egypt, the Israelites faced harsh oppression under Pharaoh's rule. A Hebrew woman from the tribe of Levi gave birth to a baby boy. Fearing for his life, she hid him for three months. But when she could hide him no longer, she made a basket from bulrushes and coated it with tar and pitch, placing the baby inside.

With a heavy heart, the mother set the basket among the reeds along the bank of the Nile River, trusting in God's protection. Meanwhile, Pharaoh's daughter came to bathe in the river and found the basket. When she saw the baby inside, she felt compassion for him and decided to adopt him as her own.

The baby's sister, watching from afar, approached Pharaoh's daughter and offered to find a Hebrew woman to nurse the child. Pharaoh's daughter agreed, and the sister brought their own mother to nurse the baby.

The baby grew and was named Moses by Pharaoh's daughter, meaning "drawn out," for she had drawn him out of the water. Moses was raised in Pharaoh's palace, but he never forgot his Hebrew heritage.

Through God's providence, Moses was spared from death and raised to become the deliverer of the Israelites. He led them out of slavery in Egypt and towards the promised land.

The story of Moses in the bulrushes teaches us about God's faithfulness and protection, even in the midst of adversity. It shows that God can use unlikely circumstances to accomplish His purposes and fulfill His plans for His people.

16. Moses and the Burning Bush

Exodus 3:1-15

In the land of Midian, Moses, once a prince of Egypt, lived as a shepherd, having fled from Pharaoh's wrath after killing an Egyptian overseer who was mistreating a Hebrew slave.

One day, as Moses led his flock to the far side of the wilderness, he came to Horeb, the mountain of God. There, he saw a remarkable sight—a bush engulfed in flames, yet it was not consumed.

Curious, Moses approached the bush, and as he drew near, God called out to him from the midst of the flames, saying, "Moses, Moses!"

Moses responded, "Here I am."

Then God said, "Do not come any closer. Take off your sandals, for the place where you are standing is holy ground. I am the God of your father, the God of Abraham, Isaac, and Jacob."

Trembling with awe and reverence, Moses hid his face, for he was afraid to look upon God.

God continued, "I have seen the suffering of my people in Egypt, and I have heard their cries. I am sending you to Pharaoh to bring my people, the Israelites, out of Egypt."

But Moses, feeling inadequate and unworthy, questioned God, saying, "Who am I that I should go to Pharaoh and bring the Israelites out of Egypt?"

God reassured Moses, saying, "I will be with you. And this will be the sign to you that it is I who have sent you: When you have brought the people out of Egypt, you will worship God on this mountain."

Encouraged by God's promise and presence, Moses accepted his calling and obeyed God's command to go to Pharaoh, setting in motion the remarkable journey of deliverance for the Israelites and the fulfillment of God's plan for His people.

17. The Plagues of Egypt

Exodus 7:14-12:30

Moses and his brother Aaron went to Pharaoh, demanding, "Let my people go, so they may worship God!" But Pharaoh hardened his heart and refused to release the Israelites from slavery.

In response, God sent a series of plagues upon the land of Egypt to demonstrate His power and persuade Pharaoh to let His people go.

The first plague was turning the waters of the Nile River into blood. The river, the source of life for Egypt, became blood, causing fish to die, and making the water undrinkable.

Despite this display of power, Pharaoh remained stubborn, refusing to heed God's warning. So, God sent a second plague—swarms of frogs that covered the land, invading homes and beds, causing great distress.

But still, Pharaoh refused to release the Israelites. And so, God sent a third plague—swarms of gnats that covered the land, tormenting the Egyptians with their bites and causing widespread discomfort.

With each subsequent refusal, God sent more plagues upon Egypt, including swarms of flies, the death of livestock, painful boils on the skin, hail mixed with fire, locusts that devoured the crops, and darkness that covered the land for three days.

Despite the devastation wrought by these plagues, Pharaoh's heart remained hardened, and he continued to resist releasing the Israelites.

Finally, God warned Pharaoh of the tenth and most severe plague—the death of the firstborn in every Egyptian household. To spare the Israelites from this judgment, God instructed them to sacrifice a lamb and smear its blood on their doorposts. When the angel of death passed over Egypt, it struck down the firstborn of every household except those marked by the blood of the lamb.

Overwhelmed by grief and fear, Pharaoh relented, and he ordered the Israelites to leave Egypt immediately. And so, the Israelites were set free from their bondage, their exodus from Egypt marking the beginning of their journey towards the promised land.

18. The Parting of the Red Sea

Exodus 14:21-31

As the Israelites fled from Egypt, Pharaoh's heart was hardened once again, and he pursued them with his army, determined to bring them back into bondage.

Trapped between the sea and Pharaoh's approaching army, the Israelites were filled with fear and cried out to Moses, "Was it because there were no graves in Egypt that you brought us to the desert to die? It would have been better for us to serve the Egyptians than to die in the desert!"

But Moses reassured the people, saying, "Do not be afraid. Stand firm and you will see the deliverance the Lord will bring you today. The Egyptians you see today you will never see again. The Lord will fight for you; you need only to be still."

Then, under God's instruction, Moses stretched out his hand over the sea, and throughout the night, the Lord drove back the sea with a strong east wind, turning the sea into dry land. The waters were divided, and the Israelites crossed through the midst of the sea on dry ground, with walls of water on their right and left.

Meanwhile, the Egyptian army pursued them into the sea, but as the morning approached, God looked down on the Egyptian army and threw it into confusion. He caused the wheels of their chariots to come off, making it impossible for them to drive.

Then, the Lord said to Moses, "Stretch out your hand over the sea so that the waters may flow back over the Egyptians and their chariots and horsemen." Moses did so, and at daybreak, the sea returned to its place, covering the entire Egyptian army that had pursued the Israelites.

Not a single one of them survived.

Witnessing the mighty power of God, the Israelites rejoiced and praised Him for delivering them from their enemies. And Moses, the servant of God, led the people in a song of thanksgiving, acknowledging God's strength and faithfulness in their time of need.

19. The Ten Commandments

Exodus 20:1-17

In the wilderness of Sinai, God summoned Moses to the top of Mount Sinai and spoke to him, saying, "I am the Lord your God, who brought you out of Egypt, out of the land of slavery."

Then God gave Moses the Ten Commandments, laying down the foundation of moral and ethical principles for His people to live by.

The first commandment was, "You shall have no other gods before me."

The second commandment was, "You shall not make for yourself an idol in the form of anything in heaven above or on the earth beneath or in the waters below."

The third commandment was, "You shall not misuse the name of the Lord your God."

The fourth commandment was, "Remember the Sabbath day by keeping it holy."

The fifth commandment was, "Honor your father and your mother."

The sixth commandment was, "You shall not murder."

The seventh commandment was, "You shall not commit adultery."

The eighth commandment was, "You shall not steal."

The ninth commandment was, "You shall not give false testimony against your neighbor."

The tenth commandment was, "You shall not covet your neighbor's house, wife, servants, animals, or anything else."

God gave these commandments to His people to guide them in righteous living and to establish the covenant relationship between Himself and the Israelites. By obeying these commandments, the people would demonstrate their love for God and their commitment to His ways, ensuring their blessings and prosperity in the land He had promised to give them.

20. The Golden Calf

Exodus 32:1-35

While Moses was on Mount Sinai receiving the Ten Commandments from God, the Israelites grew impatient and restless in their camp at the foot of the mountain.

They approached Aaron, Moses' brother, and said, "Come, make us gods who will go before us. As for this Moses, who brought us up out of Egypt, we don't know what has happened to him!"

Aaron, giving in to their demands, instructed the people to bring him their gold earrings. He melted down the gold and fashioned it into a molten calf, forming it with a tool. Then they exclaimed, "These are your gods, O Israel, who brought you up out of Egypt!"

When Aaron saw this, he built an altar in front of the calf and proclaimed, "Tomorrow there will be a festival to the Lord."

The people rose early the next day to offer burnt offerings and fellowship offerings. They sat down to eat and drink, and then indulged in revelry and debauchery.

Meanwhile, up on the mountain, God spoke to Moses, saying, "Go down, because your people, whom you brought up out of Egypt, have become corrupt. They have turned aside quickly from the way I commanded them."

Moses descended the mountain with the tablets of the covenant in his hands. When he saw the calf and the people dancing, his anger burned, and he threw the tablets down, breaking them at the foot of the mountain.

Moses confronted Aaron, demanding an explanation. Aaron shifted the blame onto the people, claiming that they were determined to do evil.

Moses then called upon those who were on the Lord's side to stand with him. The Levites rallied to him, and he instructed them to go throughout the camp, killing their brothers, friends, and neighbors who had worshiped the calf.

Afterward, Moses returned to the Lord, interceding on behalf of the people, asking for forgiveness for their great sin.

God relented from sending disaster upon the people, but the consequences of their idolatry remained.

21. Joshua and the Battle of Jericho

Joshua 6:1-27

As the Israelites prepared to enter the Promised Land, they faced their first major obstacle—the city of Jericho, a fortified city with impenetrable walls.

God spoke to Joshua, the leader of the Israelites, saying, "See, I have delivered Jericho into your hands, along with its king and its fighting men. March around the city once with all the armed men. Do this for six days. On the seventh day, march around the city seven times, with the priests blowing the trumpets. When you hear them sound a long blast on the trumpets, have the whole army give a loud shout; then the wall of the city will collapse, and the army will go up, everyone straight in."

Following God's instructions, Joshua commanded the people to march around the city of Jericho once a day for six days, with the priests carrying the ark of the covenant and blowing trumpets made of rams' horns.

On the seventh day, they marched around the city seven times, and at Joshua's command, the people shouted with a great shout. Suddenly, the walls of Jericho collapsed, and the Israelites stormed the city, capturing it and destroying everything in it—men and women, young and old, cattle, sheep, and donkeys.

Only Rahab, a prostitute who had hidden the Israelite spies, and her family were spared, as she had shown kindness to them.

The Lord was with Joshua, and his fame spread throughout the land as the Israelites continued to conquer the cities of Canaan.

The battle of Jericho serves as a testament to the power of God and His faithfulness to His promises. It demonstrates that with God on their side, the Israelites could overcome even the most formidable obstacles and inherit the land that He had promised to give them.

22. Samson and Delilah

Judges 16:4-22

Samson, a mighty judge of Israel, fell in love with a woman named Delilah, who lived in the valley of Sorek. The rulers of the Philistines approached Delilah and offered her a large sum of money if she could discover the secret of Samson's great strength.

Delilah, enticed by the offer, approached Samson and asked him, "Please tell me where your great strength lies and how you might be bound, that one could subdue you?"

Samson, initially cautious, replied with a series of false explanations, but each time Delilah tested his words, she discovered they were lies.

Finally, worn down by Delilah's persistence, Samson revealed the truth to her, saying, "No razor has ever come upon my head, for I have been a Nazirite to God from my mother's womb. If my head were shaved, then my strength would leave me, and I would become weak like any other man."

Delilah, knowing Samson's secret, conspired with the Philistine rulers to capture him. While Samson slept, she called for a man to shave off his hair, and when he awoke, his strength was gone.

The Philistines seized Samson, gouged out his eyes, and bound him in chains. They brought him to their temple to mock him, and there, between the pillars of the temple, Samson prayed to God for strength one last time.

In a final act of God's grace, Samson's strength returned to him, and he pushed against the pillars with all his might, causing the temple to collapse upon himself and the Philistines. In his death, Samson killed more Philistines than he had in his entire lifetime.

The story of Samson and Delilah serves as a cautionary tale about the consequences of giving in to temptation and revealing one's weaknesses to those who wish to harm them. It also highlights the importance of remaining faithful to God's calling and relying on His strength in times of trial.

23. David and Goliath

1 Samuel 17:1-58

In the land of Israel, the Philistines gathered their armies for battle, encamped on one hill, while the Israelites camped on another, with a valley between them.

From the Philistine camp emerged a champion named Goliath of Gath, a giant over nine feet tall, clad in armor and boasting of his strength. For forty days, Goliath challenged the Israelites to send out a champion to fight him, promising that if he defeated the Israelite champion, the Philistines would become their servants. But if the Israelite champion won, the Philistines would become the Israelites' servants.

Saul, the king of Israel, and his army were filled with fear at the sight of Goliath and his challenge. No one dared to face him.

Meanwhile, Jesse, a man from Bethlehem, sent his youngest son David to the battlefield to bring food to his brothers who were serving in Saul's army.

When David arrived at the camp and heard Goliath's taunts, he was filled with righteous indignation. He volunteered to fight Goliath, saying, "Let no one lose heart on account of this Philistine; your servant will go and fight him."

Despite Saul's doubts about David's ability to defeat Goliath, David persisted, recounting how he had killed a lion and a bear that had threatened his father's sheep, trusting in God's strength to deliver him.

Saul reluctantly agreed to let David face Goliath, and he offered David his own armor and sword. But David, unaccustomed to them, refused and instead chose five smooth stones from the brook and his sling.

As Goliath approached, David ran to meet him, slinging a stone that struck Goliath in the forehead, causing him to fall to the ground. David then took Goliath's sword and killed him, cutting off his head.

When the Philistines saw that their champion was dead, they fled in terror, and the Israelites pursued them, gaining a great victory.

David's defeat of Goliath became legendary, a testament to his faith in God's strength and his courage in the face of overwhelming odds. It also marked the beginning of David's rise to prominence as a leader and warrior in Israel.

24. David and Jonathan's Friendship

1 Samuel 18:1-4; 1 Samuel 19:1-7
1 Samuel 20:1-42

David, a young shepherd, gained fame in Israel after defeating Goliath, the Philistine champion. His courage and valor caught the attention of King Saul's son, Jonathan.

Jonathan, deeply moved by David's victory and his faith in God, formed a strong bond of friendship with him. The two men's souls were knit together, and Jonathan loved David as he loved himself.

Saul, however, became increasingly jealous of David's popularity and success. He plotted to kill David, but Jonathan, loyal to his friend, warned him of his father's plans.

Jonathan interceded on David's behalf, persuading Saul not to harm him. Despite Saul's attempts to kill David, Jonathan remained faithful to their friendship, risking his own life to protect David.

In one instance, Jonathan made a covenant with David, pledging his loyalty and promising to protect him from his father's wrath.

David and Jonathan devised a plan to test Saul's intentions. David would miss a royal feast, and if Saul showed no concern for his absence, it would confirm his desire to kill him. If Saul became angry, it would reveal his true intentions.

When Saul showed no concern for David's absence, Jonathan knew that his father's heart was set against David.

In a tearful farewell, David and Jonathan reaffirmed their friendship and made a solemn vow to each other and to their descendants.

David eventually fled from Saul's presence, but his friendship with Jonathan endured, even in their separation. Jonathan's unwavering loyalty and love for David serve as a testament to the enduring power of true friendship and the bonds of brotherhood that transcend circumstances and challenges.

25. Solomon's Wisdom

1 Kings 3:16-28

Solomon, the son of David, became king of Israel after his father's death. Early in his reign, Solomon went to Gibeon to offer sacrifices to the Lord.

One night, the Lord appeared to Solomon in a dream and said, "Ask for whatever you want me to give you."

Solomon replied, "Lord, you have shown great kindness to my father David, and now you have made me king in his place. But I am only a little child and do not know how to carry out my duties. So give your servant a discerning heart to govern your people and to distinguish between right and wrong."

Pleased with Solomon's request, the Lord said to him, "Since you have asked for this and not for long life or wealth for yourself, nor have you asked for the death of your enemies but for discernment in administering justice, I will do what you have asked. I will give you a wise and discerning heart, so that there will never have been anyone like you, nor will there ever be."

Solomon woke up and realized it was a dream. He returned to Jerusalem and stood before the Ark of the Covenant, offering burnt offerings and fellowship offerings to the Lord.

One day, two women came to Solomon, both claiming to be the mother of the same baby. They had given birth within three days of each other, but one woman's baby died during the night. Each woman insisted that the living baby was hers.

Solomon, in his wisdom, ordered a sword to be brought and commanded, "Cut the living child in two and give half to one and half to the other."

The real mother cried out, "Please, my lord, give her the living baby! Do not kill him!"

But the other woman said, "Neither I nor you shall have him. Cut him in two!"

Solomon immediately recognized the true mother's love for her child and declared, "Give the baby to the first woman. She is the real mother."

The people of Israel were amazed at Solomon's wisdom, and they feared the Lord, knowing that He had given Solomon wisdom to govern His people with justice and righteousness.

26. Solomon Builds the Temple

1 Kings 6:1-38

After David's death, his son Solomon became king of Israel. Solomon desired to honor the Lord and fulfill his father's dream of building a temple for God in Jerusalem.

In the fourth year of his reign, Solomon began the construction of the temple. He commissioned skilled craftsmen and artisans to carry out the work, using the finest materials—cedar wood from Lebanon, gold, and precious stones.

The temple was to be a magnificent structure, measuring sixty cubits long, twenty cubits wide, and thirty cubits high. It had a porch in front of the main hall, where two pillars, named Jachin and Boaz, were erected.

Inside the temple, the walls and floors were overlaid with gold, and every detail was meticulously crafted according to the Lord's instructions.

Seven years later, the temple was completed. Solomon dedicated the temple to the Lord with a great ceremony, offering sacrifices and prayers of dedication.

When Solomon prayed, the glory of the Lord filled the temple, and a cloud descended upon it, signifying God's presence among His people.

Solomon addressed the people, praising God for His faithfulness and acknowledging that the temple he had built could not contain the greatness of the Lord.

He encouraged the people to remain faithful to God's covenant and to walk in obedience to His commandments, so that they would continue to experience His blessings and protection.

The building of the temple marked a significant moment in Israel's history, symbolizing the establishment of God's dwelling place among His people and serving as a center for worship and sacrifice.

Solomon's dedication to building the temple demonstrated his reverence for the Lord and his commitment to fulfilling God's purposes. The temple stood as a lasting testimony to the glory and majesty of the God of Israel.

27. Elijah and the Widow of Zarephath

1 Kings 17:8-16

During a time when there was no rain in Israel, God spoke to the prophet Elijah, telling him to go to a town called Zarephath. God promised that a widow there would take care of him.

So, Elijah went to Zarephath. As he arrived at the town gate, he saw a widow gathering sticks. Elijah called out to her and asked for a drink of water. The widow went to get it for him.

Then Elijah asked for some bread too. The widow sadly replied that she had only a little flour and oil left. She was gathering sticks to make a final meal for herself and her son before they would die because of the drought.

But Elijah said to her, "Don't be afraid. Go home and make me a small loaf of bread first. Then make something for yourself and your son. The Lord says that your jar of flour will not run out and your jug of oil will not run dry until He sends rain again."

The widow trusted Elijah's words. She went home and did just as he had said. She made bread for Elijah, and afterward, she found that her jar of flour and jug of oil were still full, just as God had promised.

So, Elijah stayed with the widow and her son. They ate every day, and the flour and oil never ran out. God took care of them and provided for all their needs during the difficult time of drought.

28. Elijah and the Prophets of Baal

1 Kings 18:16-46

King Ahab, who ruled over Israel, had turned away from the Lord and worshiped idols, especially Baal. God sent Elijah the prophet to confront Ahab and challenge the prophets of Baal.

Elijah gathered the people of Israel and the prophets of Baal on Mount Carmel. He said to them, "How long will you waver between two opinions? If the Lord is God, follow Him; but if Baal is God, follow him."

To prove who the true God was, Elijah proposed a test. The prophets of Baal would prepare a sacrifice and call on their god to send fire to consume it, and Elijah would do the same. The god who answered by fire would be recognized as the true God.

The prophets of Baal went first. They prepared their sacrifice and called on Baal from morning until noon, dancing around the altar and shouting, but there was no response. Elijah mocked them, suggesting that perhaps Baal was sleeping or busy, or maybe he was traveling.

The prophets of Baal became more desperate, cutting themselves with swords and spears until their blood flowed, but still, there was no answer.

Then Elijah prepared his altar. He arranged the wood and the sacrifice and dug a trench around it. He poured water over the sacrifice three times, soaking the wood and filling the trench with water.

Elijah prayed to the Lord, "Answer me, Lord, so these people will know that You are God and that You are turning their hearts back again."

Immediately, fire fell from heaven, consuming the sacrifice, the wood, the stones, and even the water in the trench. The people fell prostrate, crying out, "The Lord—He is God! The Lord—He is God!"

Elijah seized the prophets of Baal and killed them, purging Israel of idolatry. The people witnessed the power of the true God, and their faith was restored.

28. Elisha Helps a Widow with Oil

2 Kings 4:1-7

There was a woman whose husband had died, and she was in trouble because she owed money to people. She went to Elisha, a man of God, and told him about her problem. She said, "My husband served the Lord, but now I have no money to pay my debts, and the people I owe are coming to take my two sons as slaves."

Elisha asked her, "What do you have in your house?"

The woman replied, "I have nothing except a small jar of olive oil."

Elisha told her, "Go and borrow as many empty jars as you can from your neighbors. Don't borrow just a few. Then go inside your house, close the door, and pour oil from your jar into all the jars you borrowed, filling each one."

The woman did as Elisha said. She gathered many empty jars, closed the door with her sons inside, and started pouring oil. To her amazement, the oil kept flowing from her small jar and filled all the other jars.

When she ran out of jars, she told her sons, and they brought her more. She kept pouring until every jar was full.

The woman went back to Elisha and told him what happened. He said to her, "Go, sell the oil, and pay your debts. You and your sons can live on what is left."

So, the woman sold the oil, paid her debts, and had enough money left over to support herself and her sons. Through Elisha's help, the widow saw a miracle where her small amount of oil was multiplied, saving her family from debt and providing for their needs.

29. Elisha and Naaman

2 Kings 5:1-19

Naaman, a mighty commander of the army of the king of Aram, was highly esteemed by his master and was a valiant warrior. However, Naaman had leprosy.

One day, a young Israelite girl who served Naaman's wife said, "If only my master would see the prophet who is in Samaria! He would cure him of his leprosy."

When Naaman heard this, he went to his master and asked for permission to go to Israel to see the prophet. The king of Aram agreed and sent Naaman with a letter to the king of Israel.

Naaman arrived in Israel with horses and chariots and stood at the door of Elisha's house. But Elisha did not come out to meet him; instead, he sent a messenger to tell Naaman, "Go, wash yourself seven times in the Jordan River, and your flesh will be restored, and you will be cleansed."

Naaman was furious. He expected Elisha to come out and perform a great miracle. Instead, he was told to wash in the Jordan River, which he considered inferior to the rivers of his own land.

But Naaman's servants convinced him to follow Elisha's instructions. So Naaman went to the Jordan River and dipped himself seven times, as Elisha had said. And miraculously, his skin was restored, and he was cleansed of his leprosy.

Overwhelmed with gratitude, Naaman returned to Elisha's house and declared, "Now I know that there is no God in all the world except in Israel. Please accept now a gift from your servant."

But Elisha refused to accept any gift from Naaman, saying, "As surely as the Lord lives, whom I serve, I will not accept a thing."

Naaman then asked for some soil from Israel to take back with him, so he could worship the Lord in his own land. He departed with a heart full of gratitude and faith in the God of Israel, whose power had healed him.

30. Jonah and the Great Fish

Jonah 1:1-17; Jonah 2:1-10

God commanded Jonah, a prophet from Israel, to go to the city of Nineveh and deliver a message of warning because of their wickedness. Instead of obeying God, Jonah decided to flee from His presence. He boarded a ship bound for Tarshish, hoping to escape God's command.

While at sea, a great storm arose, threatening to sink the ship. The sailors, fearing for their lives, cried out to their gods and cast lots to determine who was responsible for the storm. The lot fell on Jonah, and he confessed to the sailors that he was running away from the Lord.

Recognizing Jonah's connection to the storm, the sailors asked him what they should do to calm the sea. Jonah told them to throw him into the sea, and the storm would cease.

Reluctantly, the sailors threw Jonah overboard, and immediately the storm stopped. Seeing the power of

Jonah's God, the sailors feared the Lord and offered sacrifices to Him.

Meanwhile, God appointed a great fish to swallow Jonah. Inside the belly of the fish, Jonah prayed to God, acknowledging his disobedience and calling out for deliverance. He cried out to the Lord from the depths of the sea, and God heard his plea.

After three days and three nights in the belly of the fish, God commanded the fish to vomit Jonah onto dry land.

Once again, God commanded Jonah to go to Nineveh and deliver His message of warning. This time, Jonah obeyed, and he proclaimed throughout the city that in forty days, Nineveh would be overthrown because of its wickedness.

Remarkably, the people of Nineveh believed Jonah's message and repented of their sins. They declared a fast, from the greatest to the least, and put on sackcloth as a sign of their humility before God.

Witnessing Nineveh's repentance, God relented from destroying the city, showing His mercy and compassion. Jonah's reluctant obedience and God's graciousness towards Nineveh serve as a powerful reminder of God's sovereignty, mercy, and willingness to forgive those who turn to Him in repentance.

31. Esther Saves Her People

Book of Esther

Esther was a Jewish woman who lived in the Persian Empire during the time of King Xerxes. She was chosen to be queen after the previous queen disobeyed the king.

Esther's cousin, Mordecai, worked in the king's palace. One day, Mordecai overheard a plot to kill the king, and he told Esther about it. Esther told the king, and the plot was foiled.

Later, the king's advisor, Haman, became angry with Mordecai because he refused to bow down to him. Haman convinced the king to issue a decree to destroy all the Jews in the empire.

When Mordecai heard about the decree, he urged Esther to go to the king and plead for the lives of her people. Esther was scared because it was against the law to go to the king without being summoned. But Mordecai told her, "Who knows if perhaps you were made queen for such a time as this?"

Esther decided to take a risk. She fasted and prayed for three days, asking God to give her courage. Then she went to the king and invited him to a banquet.

At the banquet, Esther revealed to the king that she was Jewish and that Haman's decree meant her death as well. The king was furious, and he ordered Haman to be executed instead.

The king couldn't revoke his decree to destroy the Jews, but he issued another decree allowing the Jews to defend themselves. When the day came, the Jews fought against their enemies and were victorious.

Esther's bravery and willingness to risk her life saved her people from destruction. The Jewish people celebrated their deliverance, and Esther's story is remembered as a testament to courage, faith, and God's providence.

32. Job's Trials

Book of Job

Job was a man who lived in the land of Uz. He was wealthy, with a large family and many possessions. He was also known for his righteousness and devotion to God.

One day, Satan came before God, and God asked him if he had considered His servant Job, who was blameless and upright. Satan argued that Job only served God because he was blessed and protected. So, God allowed Satan to test Job, but He set limits on what Satan could do.

In a short span of time, Job lost everything he had. His livestock were stolen, his servants were killed, and a great wind destroyed his children's house, killing all of them.

Despite these tragedies, Job remained faithful to God. He said, "Naked I came from my mother's womb, and naked I will depart. The Lord gave and the Lord has taken away; may the name of the Lord be praised."

But Satan wasn't satisfied. He argued that Job's faithfulness was because he still had his health. So, God allowed Satan to afflict Job with painful sores all over his body.

Job's suffering was intense. He sat in ashes, scraping his sores with broken pottery. His wife urged him to curse God and die, but Job refused, saying, "Shall we accept good from God, and not trouble?"

Job's friends came to comfort him, but they ended up arguing with him, accusing him of sinning and deserving his suffering. But Job maintained his innocence and cried out to God for answers.

After a long debate, God finally spoke to Job out of a whirlwind. He didn't explain why Job had suffered, but He reminded Job of His power and wisdom. Job humbly acknowledged God's sovereignty, saying, "My ears had heard of you but now my eyes have seen you."

In the end, God restored Job's fortunes, giving him twice as much as he had before. Job's story teaches us about faithfulness in the face of suffering and the importance of trusting in God's wisdom, even when we don't understand His ways.

33. Daniel in the Lion's Den

Daniel 6:1-28

Daniel was a man who served faithfully in the kingdom of Darius the Mede. He distinguished himself with such excellence that the king planned to set him over the whole kingdom.

This stirred jealousy among the other administrators and satraps, who plotted to find grounds for charges against Daniel. But they couldn't find anything to accuse him of, as Daniel was trustworthy and neither corrupt nor negligent in his duties.

The administrators and high-ranking officials devised a plan and convinced King Darius to issue a decree that for thirty days, anyone who prayed to any god or man other than the king would be thrown into the lions' den.

Despite knowing about the decree, Daniel continued to pray three times a day to his God, just as he had done before. When the conspirators saw Daniel praying to his God, they reported him to the king.

King Darius was deeply distressed when he heard this because he valued Daniel and knew he had been tricked. However, because the law of the Medes and Persians could not be changed, he reluctantly ordered Daniel to be thrown into the lions' den.

Before Daniel was thrown in, King Darius said to him, "May your God, whom you serve continually, rescue you!"

That night, the king couldn't sleep. He was worried about Daniel and went early the next morning to the lions' den. To his relief and amazement, he found Daniel alive and unharmed. God had sent His angel to shut the mouths of the lions.

Overjoyed, King Darius ordered that Daniel be lifted out of the den. He then issued a decree that all throughout his kingdom should fear and reverence Daniel's God, "For He is the living God and He endures forever; His kingdom will not be destroyed, His dominion will never end."

Daniel's faithfulness and God's miraculous intervention in the lions' den became a testimony to the power and faithfulness of the God whom Daniel served.

34. Ezra Rebuilds the Temple

Book of Ezra

After the Babylonian exile, King Cyrus of Persia issued a decree allowing the Jews to return to Jerusalem and rebuild the temple of the Lord. Among those who returned was Ezra, a priest and scribe skilled in the Law of Moses.

Ezra led a group of exiles back to Jerusalem, carrying with them treasures that King Cyrus had entrusted to them for the temple's reconstruction. When they arrived in Jerusalem, they faced opposition from neighboring peoples who sought to hinder their efforts.

Despite these challenges, Ezra and his companions persevered. They gathered the people of Israel and began the work of rebuilding the temple. Under Ezra's leadership, they laid the foundation of the temple and began to restore it according to the instructions given by the prophets of God.

Throughout the rebuilding process, Ezra also emphasized the importance of obeying the Law of Moses and renewing the covenant with God. He taught the people the ways of the Lord and encouraged them to repent of their sins and turn back to God.

Ezra's dedication to God's Word and his leadership in the reconstruction of the temple played a crucial role in restoring the spiritual and religious life of the Jewish people in Jerusalem. Through his efforts, the temple was rebuilt, and the worship of God was reinstated in the land.

Ezra's story serves as a reminder of the importance of faithfulness to God's Word and the restoration of worship and devotion to Him. His example inspires us to remain steadfast in our commitment to God and His purposes, even in the face of challenges and opposition.

35. Nehemiah Rebuilds the Walls of Jerusalem

Book of Nehemiah

After the Babylonian exile, Nehemiah, a cupbearer to King Artaxerxes of Persia, received news about the broken walls of Jerusalem. He was deeply saddened by the state of his city and the vulnerability of its people.

Nehemiah prayed to God, asking for guidance and favor before the king. Moved by Nehemiah's distress, King Artaxerxes granted him permission to return to Jerusalem and oversee the rebuilding of the city's walls.

When Nehemiah arrived in Jerusalem, he surveyed the damage and gathered the people to share his vision of rebuilding the walls. Despite facing opposition from neighboring enemies who mocked and threatened them, Nehemiah encouraged the people to trust in God and persevere in their work.

With determination and unity, the people began the reconstruction efforts. Each family took responsibility for rebuilding a section of the wall near their own homes. They worked day and night, armed with swords and tools, ready to defend themselves against any attacks.

Nehemiah led by example, working alongside the people and offering encouragement and support. He remained steadfast in his faith in God's protection and provision throughout the rebuilding process.

Despite facing challenges and setbacks, including plots against his life and internal strife among the workers, Nehemiah remained resolute in his commitment to see the project through to completion.

After just fifty-two days of hard labor, the walls of Jerusalem were rebuilt, and the city was once again fortified and secure. The people celebrated with joy and thanksgiving, acknowledging God's faithfulness in fulfilling Nehemiah's vision and restoring the strength and dignity of Jerusalem.

Nehemiah's leadership and unwavering faith in God's promises serve as a powerful example of perseverance and trust in the face of adversity. His story inspires us to pursue God's purposes with courage and determination, knowing that He is faithful to accomplish what He has promised.

36. Jesus' Birth in Bethlehem

Luke 2:1-20

During the time of Caesar Augustus, a decree was issued that all the world should be registered. This required everyone to go to their own towns to be counted.

Joseph, a man from the town of Nazareth in Galilee, went to Bethlehem in Judea because he belonged to the house and line of David. He went there with Mary, who was pledged to be married to him and was expecting a child.

While they were in Bethlehem, the time came for the baby to be born. Mary gave birth to her firstborn, a son. She wrapped him in cloths and placed him in a manger because there was no guest room available for them.

In the fields nearby, there were shepherds keeping watch over their flocks at night. An angel of the Lord appeared to them, and the glory of the Lord shone around them. They were terrified.

But the angel said to them, "Do not be afraid. I bring you good news that will cause great joy for all the people. Today in the town of David, a Savior has been born to you; he is the Messiah, the Lord. This will be a sign to you: You will find a baby wrapped in cloths and lying in a manger."

Suddenly a great company of the heavenly host appeared with the angel, praising God and saying, "Glory to God in the highest heaven, and on earth peace to those on whom his favor rests."

When the angels had left them and gone into heaven, the shepherds hurried to Bethlehem and found Mary and Joseph, and the baby lying in the manger. After seeing him, they spread the word concerning what had been told them about this child, and all who heard it were amazed at what the shepherds said to them.

The shepherds returned, glorifying and praising God for all the things they had heard and seen, which were just as they had been told.

37. The Visit of the Wise Men

Matthew 2:1-12

After Jesus was born in Bethlehem in Judea, during the time of King Herod, Magi from the east came to Jerusalem and asked, "Where is the one who has been born king of the Jews? We saw his star when it rose and have come to worship him."

When King Herod heard this, he was disturbed, and all Jerusalem with him. He called together all the chief priests and teachers of the law and asked them where the Messiah was to be born.

"In Bethlehem in Judea," they replied, "for this is what the prophet has written: 'But you, Bethlehem, in the land of Judah, are by no means least among the rulers of Judah; for out of you will come a ruler who will shepherd my people Israel.'"

Then Herod called the Magi secretly and found out from them the exact time the star had appeared. He sent them to Bethlehem and said, "Go and search carefully for the child. As soon as you find him, report to me, so that I too may go and worship him."

After they had heard the king, they went on their way, and the star they had seen when it rose went ahead of them until it stopped over the place where the child was. When they saw the star, they were overjoyed.

On coming to the house, they saw the child with his mother Mary, and they bowed down and worshiped him. Then they opened their treasures and presented him with gifts of gold, frankincense, and myrrh.

And having been warned in a dream not to go back to Herod, they returned to their country by another route.

38. Jesus' Baptism

Matthew 3:13-17

Jesus went to the Jordan River, where John the Baptist was baptizing people. When Jesus approached John, John hesitated, saying, "I should be baptized by you, not the other way around."

But Jesus insisted, "Let it happen now, for it is right for us to do this to fulfill all righteousness."

So, John baptized Jesus. As Jesus came up out of the water, something incredible happened. The sky opened up, and the Spirit of God descended like a dove and landed on Jesus. Then, a voice from heaven said, "This is my dearly loved Son, who brings me great joy."

This was a special moment. It was the beginning of Jesus' public ministry. From this point on, Jesus would go out and teach people about God's love and forgiveness. He would heal the sick, give hope to the poor, and show everyone what it means to live a life pleasing to God.

Jesus' baptism wasn't just a ceremony. It was a significant event that marked the beginning of his mission on earth. It showed that Jesus was not just an ordinary man but the Son of God, chosen to bring salvation to the world.

Through Jesus' baptism, we also learn the importance of obedience to God's will and the significance of baptism as a symbol of our commitment to follow Jesus. Just as Jesus was baptized and received the Holy

Spirit, we too can experience the presence and power of God in our lives when we choose to follow Him wholeheartedly.

39. Jesus' Temptation in the Wilderness

Matthew 4:1-11

After Jesus was baptized, the Spirit led him into the wilderness, where he fasted for forty days and nights. During this time, the devil came to tempt him.

The devil said to Jesus, "If you are the Son of God, command these stones to become bread."

But Jesus answered, "It is written: 'Man shall not live on bread alone, but on every word that comes from the mouth of God.'"

Then, the devil took Jesus to the highest point of the temple and said, "If you are the Son of God, throw yourself down. For it is written: 'He will command his angels concerning you, and they will lift you up in their hands, so that you will not strike your foot against a stone.'"

Jesus replied, "It is also written: 'Do not put the Lord your God to the test.'"

Finally, the devil took Jesus to a very high mountain and showed him all the kingdoms of the world and their splendor. He said, "All this I will give you if you will bow down and worship me."

Jesus said to him, "Away from me, Satan! For it is written: 'Worship the Lord your God, and serve him only.'"

Then the devil left Jesus, and angels came and attended him.

In the wilderness, Jesus faced temptations that tested his faith and obedience to God. Yet, he remained steadfast, relying on the Word of God to resist the devil's schemes. This event highlights Jesus' victory over temptation and serves as an example for believers to trust in God's strength to overcome temptation in their own lives.

40. Jesus Calls His Disciples

Matthew 4:18-22; Mark 1:16-20; Luke 5:1-11

One day, as Jesus was walking along the shore of the Sea of Galilee, he saw two brothers, Simon Peter and Andrew, casting their nets into the water, for they were fishermen. Jesus called out to them, "Come, follow me, and I will make you fishers of men."

Immediately, Peter and Andrew left their nets and followed Jesus.

Further along the shore, Jesus saw two other brothers, James and John, the sons of Zebedee, in a boat with their father, mending their nets. Jesus called out to them too. Without hesitation, they left their boat and their father and followed Jesus.

From that moment on, these four fishermen became Jesus' disciples. They traveled with him, learned from him, and witnessed his teachings and miracles.

Jesus' call to his disciples was simple yet powerful. He invited them to leave behind their livelihoods and follow him, promising to teach them a new way of life. In response, Peter, Andrew, James, and John left everything behind to become followers of Jesus.

This event marks the beginning of Jesus' ministry and the formation of his inner circle of disciples. Throughout his time on earth, these men would accompany Jesus, witnessing his teachings, miracles, and ultimately, his death and resurrection.

Jesus' call to his disciples is not just a historical event but a timeless invitation for all believers to follow him. Just as Peter, Andrew, James, and John responded to Jesus' call with immediate obedience, we too are called to follow Jesus wholeheartedly, leaving behind anything that hinders us from fully embracing his teachings and way of life.

41. The Wedding at Cana

John 2:1-11

Jesus and his disciples were invited to a wedding in the town of Cana in Galilee. During the celebration, the wine ran out, which was a significant problem in Jewish culture as it could bring shame to the hosts.

Jesus' mother, Mary, approached him and said, "They have no more wine."

Jesus replied, "Woman, why do you involve me? My hour has not yet come."

However, Mary instructed the servants, "Do whatever he tells you."

Nearby, there were six stone water jars, each capable of holding twenty to thirty gallons. Jesus told the servants to fill the jars with water, and they filled them to the brim.

Then Jesus said, "Now draw some out and take it to the master of the banquet."

The servants obeyed, drawing water from the jars and taking it to the master of the banquet. When the master of the banquet tasted the water that had been turned into wine, he was astonished. He called the bridegroom over and said, "Everyone brings out the choice wine first and then the cheaper wine after the guests have had too much to drink. But you have saved the best till now!"

This, the first of his miraculous signs, Jesus performed at Cana in Galilee. He revealed his glory, and his disciples believed in him.

The wedding at Cana not only demonstrated Jesus' power to perform miracles but also his compassion and concern for the needs of others. It was a moment of joy and celebration, marking the beginning of Jesus' public ministry and the revelation of his divine nature to his disciples.

42. Jesus' Sermon on the Mount

Matthew 5:1-7:29

One day, Jesus went up on a mountainside and sat down to teach his disciples. A large crowd gathered around him, eager to hear his words.

Jesus began to teach them, saying:

"Blessed are the poor in spirit, for theirs is the kingdom of heaven.
Blessed are those who mourn, for they will be comforted.
Blessed are the meek, for they will inherit the earth.
Blessed are those who hunger and thirst for righteousness, for they will be filled.
Blessed are the merciful, for they will be shown mercy.
Blessed are the pure in heart, for they will see God.
Blessed are the peacemakers, for they will be called children of God.
Blessed are those who are persecuted because of righteousness, for theirs is the kingdom of heaven."

Jesus continued to teach the crowd, addressing various aspects of righteous living. He spoke about the importance of being salt and light in the world, loving one's enemies, and practicing forgiveness.

He also taught them how to pray, giving them the Lord's Prayer as an example. Jesus encouraged them to seek God's kingdom above all else and assured them that God would provide for their needs.

Jesus concluded his sermon by urging the crowd to enter through the narrow gate and follow the path of righteousness. He warned them against false prophets and encouraged them to build their lives on the solid foundation of his teachings.

The people were amazed at Jesus' teaching, for he spoke with authority, unlike their scribes. His sermon on the mount remains one of the most profound and influential teachings in all of history, offering timeless wisdom for righteous living and true discipleship.

43. Jesus Heals the Sick

Matthew 9:35-36

Jesus traveled throughout all the cities and villages, teaching in their synagogues, proclaiming the gospel of the kingdom, and healing every disease and sickness among the people.

When he saw the crowds, he had compassion on them, because they were harassed and helpless, like sheep without a shepherd.

Wherever Jesus went, crowds of people followed him, bringing their sick and afflicted to be healed. They brought the blind, the lame, the deaf, and those possessed by demons. And Jesus healed them all.

He touched the blind, and they received their sight. He spoke to the lame, and they walked again. He commanded the deaf to hear, and their ears were opened. And those tormented by demons were set free by his word.

Word of Jesus' miraculous healings spread far and wide, and people from all over came to see him. They brought their sick loved ones, hoping that they too would receive healing at the hands of Jesus.

Jesus' ministry of healing was a powerful demonstration of God's compassion and mercy toward the suffering and afflicted. It showed his authority over sickness and disease and foreshadowed the ultimate healing and restoration he would bring through his death and resurrection.

Through Jesus' healing miracles, many came to believe in him as the Son of God and the promised Messiah. His ministry brought hope to the hopeless and comfort to the suffering, revealing God's love for all humanity and his desire to bring wholeness and restoration to every aspect of our lives.

44. Jesus Raises Lazarus from the Dead

John 11:1-44

In the town of Bethany, there lived a man named Lazarus, who was the brother of Mary and Martha. Lazarus fell ill, and his sisters sent word to Jesus, saying, "Lord, the one you love is sick."

When Jesus heard this, he said, "This sickness will not end in death. No, it is for God's glory so that God's Son may be glorified through it."

Though he loved Lazarus and his sisters, Jesus stayed where he was for two more days. Then, he said to his disciples, "Let us go back to Judea."

When Jesus arrived in Bethany, Lazarus had already been in the tomb for four days. Martha went out to meet Jesus, and she said to him, "Lord, if you had been here, my brother would not have died."

Jesus comforted Martha, saying, "Your brother will rise again."

Martha replied, "I know he will rise again in the resurrection at the last day."

Jesus said to her, "I am the resurrection and the life. The one who believes in me will live, even though they die; and whoever lives by believing in me will never die. Do you believe this?"

Martha answered, "Yes, Lord. I believe that you are the Messiah, the Son of God, who is to come into the world."

Jesus then went to the tomb, which was a cave with a stone laid across the entrance. He asked that the stone be removed, and then he prayed to his Father in heaven.

After praying, Jesus called out in a loud voice, "Lazarus, come out!"

To the amazement of all who were present, Lazarus emerged from the tomb, still wrapped in burial cloths.

Jesus said to them, "Take off the grave clothes and let him go."

This miraculous event caused many who witnessed it to believe in Jesus as the Son of God, the giver of life, and the one who has power even over death itself.

45. Jesus Feeds the Five Thousand

Matthew 14:13-21; Mark 6:30-44 Luke 9:10-17; John 6:1-15

One day, Jesus withdrew to a remote place to be alone with his disciples after hearing about the death of John the Baptist. However, a large crowd followed them, eager to hear Jesus teach and to see the miracles he performed.

Seeing the multitude, Jesus had compassion on them and began to teach them many things about the kingdom of God. As evening approached, the disciples came to Jesus and suggested that he send the people away so they could find food in the nearby villages.

But Jesus said to them, "They do not need to go away. You give them something to eat."

The disciples were surprised and replied, "We have only five loaves of bread and two fish, unless we go and buy food for all these people."

Jesus instructed the disciples to bring him the loaves and fish. Then, he took the bread, gave thanks, and broke it. He also did the same with the fish. Afterward, he distributed the food to the crowds through his disciples.

Miraculously, everyone ate and was satisfied. Not only did the five thousand men (plus women and children) eat their fill, but there were also twelve baskets of leftovers collected afterward.

This miraculous feeding demonstrated Jesus' power and provision. He showed compassion for the hungry crowd and met their physical needs in an extraordinary way. The event also served as a sign of Jesus' identity as the Messiah, who fulfills the promises of God to provide for his people abundantly.

The feeding of the five thousand remains one of the most well-known and significant miracles performed by

Jesus during his earthly ministry, illustrating his compassion, power, and ability to meet the needs of all who come to him in faith.

46. Jesus Walks on Water

Matthew 14:22-33; Mark 6:45-52
John 6:16-21

After feeding the five thousand, Jesus made his disciples get into a boat and go ahead of him to the other side of the Sea of Galilee, while he dismissed the crowd. Afterward, Jesus went up on a mountainside to pray alone.

As evening approached, the disciples found themselves in the middle of the sea, struggling against strong winds and waves. Jesus saw them from the mountainside and, in the fourth watch of the night, came to them, walking on the surface of the water.

When the disciples saw Jesus walking on the water, they were terrified, thinking he was a ghost. But Jesus reassured them, saying, "Take courage! It is I. Don't be afraid."

Peter, filled with faith, responded, "Lord, if it's you, tell me to come to you on the water."

"Come," Jesus said.

So, Peter got out of the boat and walked on the water toward Jesus. But when he saw the wind, he was afraid and began to sink. He cried out, "Lord, save me!"

Immediately, Jesus reached out his hand and caught Peter. He said, "You of little faith, why did you doubt?"

When Jesus and Peter climbed into the boat, the wind died down, and the disciples worshiped him, saying, "Truly you are the Son of God!"

This miraculous event demonstrated Jesus' authority over nature and his ability to provide comfort and security to his disciples in times of fear and uncertainty. It also challenged Peter to have faith and trust in Jesus, even in the midst of life's storms.

Through walking on water, Jesus revealed his divine nature and power, showing that he is the one who can calm the storms of life and lead us safely through any situation when we put our trust in him.

47. The Transfiguration of Jesus

Matthew 17:1-13; Mark 9:2-13; Luke 9:28-36

Jesus took Peter, James, and John, his closest disciples, and led them up a high mountain to pray. As Jesus prayed, his appearance changed before them. His face shone like the sun, and his clothes became as white as light.

Suddenly, Moses and Elijah appeared and began talking with Jesus. Peter, filled with awe and excitement, said to Jesus, "Lord, it is good for us to be here. If you wish, I will put up three shelters—one for you, one for Moses, and one for Elijah."

While Peter was still speaking, a bright cloud enveloped them, and a voice from the cloud said, "This is my Son, whom I love; with him I am well pleased. Listen to him!"

When the disciples heard this, they fell facedown to the ground, terrified. But Jesus came and touched them. "Get up," he said. "Don't be afraid." When they looked up, they saw no one except Jesus.

As they descended the mountain, Jesus instructed them, "Don't tell anyone what you have seen until the Son of Man has been raised from the dead."

The disciples were confused and wondered what Jesus meant by "raised from the dead." They kept this vision to themselves, discussing among themselves what "raised from the dead" might mean.

The transfiguration of Jesus revealed his divine glory to Peter, James, and John, giving them a glimpse of his true nature as the Son of God. It also affirmed the continuity between Jesus and the Old Testament prophets, symbolized by the presence of Moses and Elijah.

This extraordinary event strengthened the disciples' faith and prepared them for the challenges that lay ahead, reminding them to listen to Jesus and trust in his authority as the beloved Son of God.

48. Jesus' Triumphal Entry into Jerusalem

Matthew 21:1-11; Mark 11:1-11 Luke 19:28-44; John 12:12-19

As Jesus approached Jerusalem, he sent two of his disciples ahead, saying to them, "Go to the village ahead of you, and as you enter it, you will find a colt tied there, which no one has ever ridden. Untie it and bring it here. If anyone asks you why you are untying it, say, 'The Lord needs it.'"

The disciples did as Jesus instructed, and they found the colt, just as he had said. As they were untying the colt, its owners asked them what they were doing. The disciples replied as Jesus had told them, and the owners allowed them to take the colt.

They brought the colt to Jesus and threw their cloaks over it. Jesus sat on the colt, and as he rode toward Jerusalem, a large crowd spread their cloaks on the road, while others cut branches from the trees and spread them on the road ahead.

The crowds that went ahead of him and those that followed shouted, "Hosanna to the Son of David! Blessed is he who comes in the name of the Lord! Hosanna in the highest heaven!"

The whole city was stirred and asked, "Who is this?"

The crowds answered, "This is Jesus, the prophet from Nazareth in Galilee!"

As Jesus entered Jerusalem, the city was filled with excitement and anticipation. The people hailed him as their long-awaited Messiah, the one who would bring salvation and deliverance to Israel.

However, Jesus knew the true reason for his entry into Jerusalem. He knew that he was fulfilling prophecy and that his ultimate purpose was to offer himself as the sacrificial Lamb of God for the sins of the world.

The triumphal entry into Jerusalem marked the beginning of Jesus' final week on earth, leading up to his crucifixion and resurrection. It was a moment of both celebration and solemnity, as Jesus willingly embarked on the path that would ultimately lead to the redemption of humanity.

49. The Last Supper

Matthew 26:17-30; Mark 14:12-26
Luke 22:7-38; John 13:1-17:26

As the Passover feast approached, Jesus instructed his disciples to go into the city, where they would meet a man carrying a jar of water. They were to follow him to a house, where they would prepare for the Passover meal.

That evening, Jesus and his twelve disciples gathered in the upper room of the house to share the Passover meal. As they reclined at the table, Jesus said to them, "I have eagerly desired to eat this Passover with you before I suffer. For I tell you, I will not eat it again until it finds fulfillment in the kingdom of God."

During the meal, Jesus took bread, gave thanks, and broke it, saying, "This is my body, given for you; do this in remembrance of me." Then he took a cup, gave thanks, and said, "This cup is the new covenant in my blood, which is poured out for you."

As they ate, Jesus told his disciples that one of them would betray him. This troubled the disciples, and each one asked, "Surely you don't mean me, Lord?"

Jesus replied, "The one who has dipped his hand into the bowl with me will betray me. The Son of Man will go just as it is written about him. But woe to that man who betrays the Son of Man! It would be better for him if he had not been born."

Then Judas Iscariot, one of the twelve disciples, left the room to betray Jesus to the religious authorities.

After Judas had gone, Jesus continued to teach and comfort his disciples. He washed their feet as a symbol of humble service and love, instructing them to do likewise for one another.

The Last Supper was a significant moment in Jesus' ministry, as he shared his final meal with his closest followers and instituted the sacrament of communion. It foreshadowed his impending sacrifice on the cross and served as a powerful symbol of his love and redemption for all who would believe in him.

50. Jesus Prays in Gethsemane

Matthew 26:36-46; Mark 14:32-42; Luke 22:39-46

After the Last Supper, Jesus went with his disciples to the Garden of Gethsemane, a place he often visited for prayer. He said to them, "Sit here while I go over there and pray."

Taking Peter, James, and John with him, Jesus began to feel deeply distressed and troubled. He said to them, "My soul is overwhelmed with sorrow to the point of death. Stay here and keep watch with me."

Going a little farther, Jesus fell with his face to the ground and prayed, "Father, if it is possible, may this cup be taken from me. Yet not as I will, but as you will."

An angel from heaven appeared to him and strengthened him. Being in anguish, Jesus prayed more earnestly, and his sweat was like drops of blood falling to the ground.

Returning to his disciples, Jesus found them sleeping and said, "Couldn't you men keep watch with me for one hour? Watch and pray so that you will not fall into temptation. The spirit is willing, but the flesh is weak."

Once again, Jesus went away and prayed the same thing. When he returned, he found them sleeping again because their eyes were heavy.

Leaving them once more, Jesus prayed the third time, saying the same thing. Then he returned to his disciples and said to them, "Are you still sleeping and resting? Look, the hour has come, and the Son of Man is delivered into the hands of sinners. Rise! Let us go! Here comes my betrayer!"

In the garden of Gethsemane, Jesus experienced intense emotional and spiritual agony as he faced the impending suffering and death that awaited him on the cross. His prayer to the Father revealed his humanity, yet his submission to God's will demonstrated his obedience and ultimate sacrifice for the redemption of humanity.

51. Jesus' Trial before Pilate

Matthew 27:11-26; Mark 15:1-15; Luke 23:1-25; John 18:28-19:16

After Jesus was arrested in the Garden of Gethsemane, he was brought before the Roman governor, Pontius Pilate, to be tried.

The religious leaders of the Jewish Sanhedrin accused Jesus of blasphemy and claimed that he was a threat to the Roman Empire. They demanded that Pilate sentence Jesus to death.

Pilate questioned Jesus, asking him if he was the king of the Jews. Jesus replied, "You say so," but he did not defend himself against the false accusations.

Pilate was amazed by Jesus' silence and innocence. He tried to release Jesus, knowing that he had done nothing deserving of death. However, the crowd, stirred up by the religious leaders, shouted, "Crucify him!"

Pilate, wanting to satisfy the crowd and maintain peace, handed Jesus over to be crucified. He washed his hands in front of the crowd, saying, "I am innocent of this man's blood. It is your responsibility."

Despite knowing Jesus' innocence, Pilate gave in to the pressure of the crowd and ordered that Jesus be flogged and crucified.

Jesus' trial before Pilate highlights the injustice and corruption of human authorities. Although Pilate knew that Jesus was innocent, he chose to prioritize his own interests and political ambitions over justice and righteousness.

Ultimately, Jesus' trial before Pilate fulfilled the prophecy of his suffering and death, demonstrating his willingness to endure unjust condemnation and humiliation for the sake of humanity's salvation. Through his sacrificial death on the cross, Jesus atoned for the sins of the world and offered forgiveness and redemption to all who believe in him.

52. The Crucifixion of Jesus

Matthew 27:32-56; Mark 15:21-41; Luke 23:26-49; John 19:16-37

After Jesus was sentenced to death by Pontius Pilate, the Roman soldiers led him away to be crucified. They forced a man named Simon of Cyrene to carry Jesus' cross to the place called Golgotha, meaning "Place of the Skull."

At Golgotha, they nailed Jesus to the cross, along with two criminals, one on each side of him. Above Jesus' head, Pilate had a sign attached that read, "Jesus of Nazareth, the King of the Jews," written in Hebrew, Latin, and Greek.

As Jesus hung on the cross, people passing by hurled insults at him, mocking him and challenging him to save himself if he truly was the Son of God. Even the religious leaders and soldiers mocked him, saying, "He saved others, but he can't save himself! Let him come down from the cross, and then we will believe in him."

One of the criminals crucified with Jesus also taunted him, but the other criminal rebuked him, saying, "Don't you fear God? We are being punished justly, for we are getting what our deeds deserve. But this man has done nothing wrong." Then he said to Jesus, "Remember me when you come into your kingdom."

Jesus replied, "Truly I tell you, today you will be with me in paradise."

As Jesus hung on the cross, darkness came over the whole land for three hours, from noon until three in the afternoon. Then Jesus cried out in a loud voice, "My God, my God, why have you forsaken me?" He then said, "It is finished," and he breathed his last.

At that moment, the earth shook, the rocks split, and the curtain of the temple was torn in two from top to bottom. Seeing these signs, the centurion and those with him realized that Jesus was indeed the Son of God.

The crucifixion of Jesus is the central event of Christian faith, representing the sacrificial love of God and the atonement for humanity's sins. Through his death on the cross, Jesus provided the way for salvation and reconciliation between God and humanity.

53. Jesus' Resurrection

Matthew 28:1-20; Mark 16:1-20; Luke 24:1-53; John 20:1-31

After Jesus was crucified and buried, on the third day, which was the first day of the week, Mary Magdalene and the other Mary went to the tomb.

Suddenly, there was a great earthquake, for an angel of the Lord descended from heaven, rolled back the stone from the entrance, and sat on it. His appearance was like lightning, and his clothes were as white as snow.

The guards were so afraid that they shook and became like dead men. But the angel said to the women, "Do not be afraid, for I know that you are looking for Jesus, who was crucified. He is not here; he has risen, just as he said. Come and see the place where he lay. Then go quickly and tell his disciples: 'He has risen from the dead and is going ahead of you into Galilee. There you will see him.' Now I have told you."

The women hurried away from the tomb, afraid yet filled with joy, and ran to tell his disciples. Suddenly, Jesus met them. "Greetings," he said. They came to him, clasped his feet, and worshiped him.

Then Jesus said to them, "Do not be afraid. Go and tell my brothers to go to Galilee; there they will see me."

Meanwhile, the guards went into the city and reported to the chief priests everything that had happened. When the chief priests had met with the elders and devised a plan, they gave the soldiers a large sum of money, telling them, "You are to say, 'His disciples came during the night and stole him away while we were asleep.' If this report gets to the governor, we will satisfy him and keep you out of trouble."

So, the soldiers took the money and did as they were instructed. And this story has been widely circulated among the Jews to this very day.

The resurrection of Jesus marks his victory over sin and death. It is the foundation of Christian faith, providing hope for believers and demonstrating God's power to overcome even the greatest obstacles.

54. The Road to Emmaus

Luke 24:13-35

On the day of Jesus' resurrection, two of his disciples were walking from Jerusalem to Emmaus, a village about seven miles away. As they walked, they talked about everything that had happened in Jerusalem, including Jesus' crucifixion and the reports of his resurrection.

As they were discussing these things, Jesus himself came up and walked along with them, but they were kept from recognizing him. He asked them, "What are you discussing together as you walk along?"

They stood still, their faces downcast. One of them, named Cleopas, asked him, "Are you the only one visiting Jerusalem who does not know the things that have happened there in these days?"

"What things?" Jesus asked.

They replied, "About Jesus of Nazareth. He was a prophet, powerful in word and deed before God and all the people. The chief priests and our rulers handed him over to be sentenced to death, and they crucified him. But we had hoped that he was the one who was going to redeem Israel. And what is more, it is the third day since all this took place. Some of our women amazed us; they went to the tomb early this morning but didn't find his body. They came and told us that they had seen a vision of angels, who said he was alive. Then some of our companions went to the tomb and found it just as the women had said, but they did not see Jesus."

Jesus said to them, "How foolish you are, and how slow to believe all that the prophets have spoken! Did not the Messiah have to suffer these things and then enter his glory?" And beginning with Moses and all the Prophets, he explained to them what was said in all the Scriptures concerning himself.

As they approached the village, Jesus continued on as if he were going farther. But they urged him strongly, "Stay with us, for it is nearly evening; the day is almost over." So, he went in to stay with them.

When he was at the table with them, he took bread, gave thanks, broke it, and began to give it to them. Then their eyes were opened, and they recognized him, and he disappeared from their sight.

They asked each other, "Were not our hearts burning within us while he talked with us on the road and opened the Scriptures to us?"

They got up and returned at once to Jerusalem. There they found the Eleven and those with them, assembled together and saying, "It is true! The Lord has risen and has appeared to Simon." Then the two told what had happened on the way, and how Jesus was recognized by them when he broke the bread.

The encounter on the road to Emmaus is a beautiful illustration of Jesus' post-resurrection appearances and his ability to open the Scriptures to reveal himself. It shows how Jesus can transform despair into hope and confusion into understanding through his presence and teaching.

55. Jesus Appears to His Disciples

John 20:19-29

On the evening of the first day of the week, the disciples were together, with the doors locked for fear of the Jewish leaders. Suddenly, Jesus came and stood among them and said, "Peace be with you!"

After he said this, he showed them his hands and side. The disciples were overjoyed when they saw the Lord.

Again, Jesus said, "Peace be with you! As the Father has sent me, I am sending you." And with that, he breathed on them and said, "Receive the Holy Spirit. If you forgive anyone's sins, their sins are forgiven; if you do not forgive them, they are not forgiven."

Now Thomas, one of the Twelve, was not with the disciples when Jesus came. So, the other disciples told him, "We have seen the Lord!"

But he said to them, "Unless I see the nail marks in his hands and put my finger where the nails were, and put my hand into his side, I will not believe."

A week later, Jesus' disciples were in the house again, and Thomas was with them. Though the doors were locked, Jesus came and stood among them and said, "Peace be with you!"

Then he said to Thomas, "Put your finger here; see my hands. Reach out your hand and put it into my side. Stop doubting and believe."

Thomas said to him, "My Lord and my God!"

Then Jesus told him, "Because you have seen me, you have believed; blessed are those who have not seen and yet have believed."

Jesus' appearance to his disciples demonstrates his victory over death and his ability to overcome barriers, such as locked doors, to bring peace and assurance to his followers. It also emphasizes the importance of faith and belief, even in the absence of physical evidence, as Jesus commends those who believe without seeing.

56. The Great Commission

Matthew 28:16-20

After Jesus rose from the dead, he appeared to his disciples in Galilee, where he had instructed them to meet him. When they saw him, they worshiped him, but some were still unsure.

Jesus approached them and said, "All authority in heaven and on earth has been given to me. So, go and make disciples of all nations. Baptize them in the name of the Father, the Son, and the Holy Spirit. Teach them to obey everything I have commanded you."

He assured them, "I will be with you always, even until the end of the age."

The disciples listened intently to Jesus' words. They understood that he was entrusting them with an important mission—to spread the message of God's love and salvation to people everywhere.

With newfound determination, the disciples set out to fulfill the Great Commission. They traveled far and wide, sharing the good news of Jesus' resurrection and inviting others to follow him.

They baptized new believers and taught them the ways of Jesus, showing them how to love God and love one another. They faced many challenges along the way, but they were encouraged by Jesus' promise to be with them always.

As they obeyed Jesus' command, the disciples saw countless lives transformed by the power of the gospel. People from every nation came to know Jesus as their Lord and Savior, and communities were changed for the better.

The Great Commission wasn't just for the disciples—it's a calling for all believers, even today. Jesus' words remind us that we have a responsibility to share his love with others and to make disciples wherever we go. And just like the disciples, we can trust that Jesus is always with us, guiding and empowering us as we carry out his mission.

57. Pentecost

Acts 2:1-13

After Jesus ascended to heaven, his disciples gathered together in Jerusalem. They were waiting as Jesus had instructed them to do for the Holy Spirit to come upon them.

Suddenly, a sound like a mighty rushing wind filled the entire house where they were sitting. Then, something that looked like tongues of fire appeared and settled on each of them. They were all filled with the Holy Spirit and began to speak in other languages, as the Spirit enabled them.

Now, there were devout Jews from every nation under heaven staying in Jerusalem. When they heard the sound, a crowd gathered, bewildered because each one heard the disciples speaking in their own language. They were amazed and asked, "Aren't all these who are speaking Galileans? How then is it that each of us hears them in our native language? Parthians, Medes, and Elamites; residents of Mesopotamia, Judea, and Cappadocia, Pontus and Asia, Phrygia and Pamphylia, Egypt and the parts of Libya near Cyrene; visitors from Rome (both Jews and converts to Judaism); Cretans and Arabs—we hear them declaring the wonders of God in our own tongues!"

They were all astonished and perplexed, wondering what this meant. Some, however, mocked and said, "They have had too much wine."

But Peter, standing up with the eleven, raised his voice and addressed the crowd, explaining that what was happening was the fulfillment of prophecy spoken by the prophet Joel. He urged them to repent and be baptized in the name of Jesus Christ for the forgiveness of their sins, promising that they too would receive the gift of the Holy Spirit.

Pentecost marked the outpouring of the Holy Spirit upon the disciples, empowering them to boldly proclaim the gospel to people of all nations and languages. It was the birth of the Christian church, as thousands of people responded to Peter's message and were baptized, beginning a new era of faith and salvation in Jesus Christ.

58. Peter and John Heal a Beggar

Acts 3:1-10

One day, Peter and John went to the temple at the time of prayer. As they approached the temple gate called Beautiful, they saw a man who had been lame from birth. He was being carried to the temple gate to beg for money from those going into the temple courts.

When he saw Peter and John about to enter, he asked them for money. Peter looked straight at him, as did John. Then Peter said, "Look at us!" So the man gave them his attention, expecting to receive something from them.

But Peter said, "Silver or gold I do not have, but what I do have I give you. In the name of Jesus Christ of Nazareth, walk." Taking him by the right hand, he helped him up, and instantly the man's feet and ankles became strong. He jumped to his feet and began to walk. Then he went with them into the temple courts, walking and jumping, and praising God.

When all the people saw him walking and praising God, they recognized him as the same man who used to sit begging at the temple gate called Beautiful, and they were filled with wonder and amazement at what had happened to him.

The healing of the lame beggar by Peter and John demonstrated the power of Jesus' name and the authority given to his followers. It was a miraculous sign that attracted attention and opened the hearts of many to believe in Jesus as the Messiah. The beggar's transformation from helplessness to joyous praise glorified God and served as a powerful testimony to the reality of Jesus' resurrection and the ongoing work of his Spirit in the world.

59. Ananias and Sapphira

Acts 5:1-11

In the early days of the Christian church, there were great signs and wonders performed by the apostles. The believers were of one heart and mind, sharing everything they had.

Now, a man named Ananias, together with his wife Sapphira, sold a piece of property. With his wife's full knowledge, he kept back part of the money for himself, but brought the rest and put it at the apostles' feet.

Then Peter said, "Ananias, how is it that Satan has so filled your heart that you have lied to the Holy Spirit and have kept for yourself some of the money you received for the land? Didn't it belong to you before it was sold? And after it was sold, wasn't the money at your disposal? What made you think of doing such a thing? You have not lied just to human beings but to God."

When Ananias heard this, he fell down and died. And great fear seized all who heard what had happened.

Then some young men came forward, wrapped up his body, and carried him out and buried him.

About three hours later, his wife came in, not knowing what had happened. Peter asked her, "Tell me, is this the price you and Ananias got for the land?"

"Yes," she said, "that is the price."

Peter said to her, "How could you conspire to test the Spirit of the Lord? Listen! The feet of the men who buried your husband are at the door, and they will carry you out also."

At that moment, she fell down at his feet and died. Then the young men came in and, finding her dead, carried her out and buried her beside her husband.

The story of Ananias and Sapphira serves as a sobering reminder of the importance of honesty and integrity before God. Their deception and greed brought swift judgment upon them, highlighting the seriousness of sin and the need for sincerity and truthfulness in all our dealings.

60. Philip and the Ethiopian Eunuch

Acts 8:26-40

One day, an angel of the Lord said to Philip, "Go south to the road—the desert road—that goes down from Jerusalem to Gaza." So he started out on his journey.

As he traveled along the road, he met an Ethiopian eunuch, an important official in charge of all the treasury of the Kandake (which means "queen of the Ethiopians"). The eunuch had gone to Jerusalem to worship and was now on his way home. He was sitting in his chariot, reading the Book of Isaiah.

The Spirit told Philip, "Go to that chariot and stay near it."

Philip ran up to the chariot and heard the man reading aloud from the Book of Isaiah. "Do you understand what you are reading?" Philip asked.

The eunuch replied, "How can I, unless someone explains it to me?" So he invited Philip to come up and sit with him.

The eunuch was reading this passage of Scripture:

"He was led like a sheep to the slaughter,
   and as a lamb before its shearer is silent,
   so he did not open his mouth.
In his humiliation he was deprived of justice.
   Who can speak of his descendants?
   For his life was taken from the earth."

The eunuch asked Philip, "Tell me, please, who is the prophet talking about, himself or someone else?"

Then Philip began with that very passage of Scripture and told him the good news about Jesus.

As they traveled along the road, they came to some water and the eunuch said, "Look, here is water. What can stand in the way of my being baptized?" So he gave orders to stop the chariot. Then both Philip and the eunuch went down into the water and Philip baptized him.

When they came up out of the water, the Spirit of the Lord suddenly took Philip away, and the eunuch did not see him again, but went on his way rejoicing.

The encounter between Philip and the Ethiopian eunuch demonstrates God's sovereign orchestration of divine appointments and his desire for all people to hear and respond to the gospel message. Philip's obedience to the Spirit's leading resulted in the salvation of the eunuch, who eagerly received the good news of Jesus Christ and was baptized, illustrating the inclusive nature of God's kingdom and the power of the gospel to transform lives.

61. Paul's Conversion on the Road to Damascus

Acts 9:1-19

Saul, a devout Pharisee, was on his way to Damascus with official letters authorizing him to arrest followers of Jesus. Suddenly, a light from heaven flashed around him. He fell to the ground and heard a voice say to him, "Saul, Saul, why do you persecute me?"

"Who are you, Lord?" Saul asked.

"I am Jesus, whom you are persecuting," he replied. "Now get up and go into the city, and you will be told what you must do."

The men traveling with Saul stood there speechless; they heard the sound but did not see anyone. Saul got up from the ground, but when he opened his eyes, he could see nothing. So, they led him by the hand into Damascus.

For three days, Saul was blind and did not eat or drink anything. In Damascus, there was a disciple named Ananias. The Lord called to him in a vision, "Ananias!"

"Yes, Lord," he answered.

The Lord told him, "Go to the house of Judas on Straight Street and ask for a man from Tarsus named Saul, for he is praying. In a vision, he has seen a man named Ananias come and place his hands on him to restore his sight."

Ananias protested, knowing Saul's reputation as a persecutor of the church. But the Lord reassured him, saying, "Go! This man is my chosen instrument to proclaim my name to the Gentiles and their kings and to the people of Israel."

So, Ananias went to the house where Saul was staying. Placing his hands on Saul, he said, "Brother Saul, the Lord—Jesus, who appeared to you on the road as you were coming here—has sent me so that you may see again and be filled with the Holy Spirit."

Immediately, something like scales fell from Saul's eyes, and he could see again. He got up and was baptized. After taking some food, he regained his strength.

Saul's encounter with Jesus on the road to Damascus marked the beginning of his transformation from a persecutor of Christians to one of the greatest apostles of the early church. His conversion illustrates the power of God to change hearts and lives, even those who seem least likely to turn to him.

Certainly! Here's the revised story with the addition of the name change information at the end:

62. Paul's Conversion on the Road to Damascus

Acts 9:1-19

Saul, a devout Pharisee, was on his way to Damascus with official letters authorizing him to arrest followers of Jesus. Suddenly, a light from heaven flashed around him. He fell to the ground and heard a voice say to him, "Saul, Saul, why do you persecute me?"

"Who are you, Lord?" Saul asked.

"I am Jesus, whom you are persecuting," he replied. "Now get up and go into the city, and you will be told what you must do."

The men traveling with Saul stood there speechless; they heard the sound but did not see anyone. Saul got up from the ground, but when he opened his eyes, he could see nothing. So, they led him by the hand into Damascus.

For three days, Saul was blind and did not eat or drink anything. In Damascus, there was a disciple named Ananias. The Lord called to him in a vision, "Ananias!"

"Yes, Lord," he answered.

The Lord told him, "Go to the house of Judas on Straight Street and ask for a man from Tarsus named Saul, for he is praying. In a vision, he has seen a man named Ananias come and place his hands on him to restore his sight."

Ananias protested, knowing Saul's reputation as a persecutor of the church. But the Lord reassured him, saying, "Go! This man is my chosen instrument to proclaim my name to the Gentiles and their kings and to the people of Israel."

So, Ananias went to the house where Saul was staying. Placing his hands on Saul, he said, "Brother Saul, the Lord—Jesus, who appeared to you on the road as you were coming here—has sent me so that you may see again and be filled with the Holy Spirit."

Immediately, something like scales fell from Saul's eyes, and he could see again. He got up and was baptized. After taking some food, he regained his strength.

Saul's encounter with Jesus on the road to Damascus marked the beginning of his transformation from a persecutor of Christians to one of the greatest apostles of the early church. Following this experience, Saul, also known as Paul, became instrumental in spreading the gospel throughout the Gentile world, enduring hardships and persecution for the sake of Christ.

63. Paul and Barnabas in Antioch

Acts 11:19-30

In the city of Antioch, some believers who had been scattered by persecution began preaching the word about Jesus, not only to Jews but also to Gentiles.

When news of this reached the church in Jerusalem, they sent Barnabas to Antioch. He saw the grace of God at work among the believers and encouraged them to remain true to the Lord with all their hearts.

Barnabas then went to Tarsus to look for Saul. When he found him, he brought him back to Antioch. For a whole year, Barnabas and Saul met with the church and taught great numbers of people. It was in Antioch that the disciples were first called Christians.

During this time, some prophets came down from Jerusalem to Antioch. One of them, named Agabus, stood up and through the Spirit predicted a severe famine that would spread over the entire Roman world. This famine occurred during the reign of Claudius.

The disciples in Antioch decided to provide help for the brothers and sisters living in Judea, each according to their ability. They sent their gift to the elders by Barnabas and Saul.

Paul and Barnabas's ministry in Antioch demonstrated the transformative power of the gospel to unite people from diverse backgrounds into one faith community. Their teaching and encouragement strengthened believers and laid the groundwork for further missionary endeavors. Additionally, the generous response of the Antiochian believers to the needs of their brothers and sisters in Judea exemplified the spirit of love and solidarity within the early church.

64. Paul and Barnabas in Antioch

Acts 11:19-26

In the city of Antioch, after the persecution that arose over Stephen, some believers traveled as far as Phoenicia, Cyprus, and Antioch, preaching the word to no one but Jews. But there were some of them, men of Cyprus and Cyrene, who, on coming to Antioch, spoke to the Hellenists also, preaching the Lord Jesus. And the hand of the Lord was with them, and a great number who believed turned to the Lord.

The news of these events reached the ears of the church in Jerusalem, and they sent Barnabas to Antioch. When he came and saw the grace of God, he was glad, and he exhorted them all to remain faithful to the Lord with steadfast purpose, for he was a good man, full of the Holy Spirit and of faith. And a great many people were added to the Lord.

So Barnabas went to Tarsus to look for Saul, and when he had found him, he brought him to Antioch. For a whole year they met with the church and taught a great many people. And in Antioch the disciples were first called Christians.

During this time, prophets came down from Jerusalem to Antioch. One of them named Agabus stood up and foretold by the Spirit that there would be a great famine over all the world; this took place in the days of Claudius. So the disciples determined, every one according to his ability, to send relief to the brothers living in Judea. And they did so, sending it to the elders by the hand of Barnabas and Saul.

Paul and Barnabas's ministry in Antioch showcased the inclusive nature of the gospel, reaching both Jews and Gentiles. Their teaching and leadership led to the growth of the church and the emergence of the term "Christians" for the followers of Jesus. Additionally, the church's response to the impending famine demonstrated their commitment to supporting fellow believers in times of need.

65. Paul and Silas in Prison

Acts 16:16-40

While Paul and Silas were in the city of Philippi, a slave girl possessed by a spirit of divination followed them, shouting, "These men are servants of the Most High God, who are telling you the way to be saved." This she kept up for many days. Finally, Paul became so annoyed that he turned around and said to the spirit, "In the name of Jesus Christ I command you to come out of her!" At that moment the spirit left her.

When her owners realized that their hope of making money was gone, they seized Paul and Silas and dragged them into the marketplace to face the authorities. They brought them before the magistrates and said, "These men are Jews, and are throwing our city into an uproar by advocating customs unlawful for us Romans to accept or practice."

The crowd joined in the attack against Paul and Silas, and the magistrates ordered them to be stripped and beaten with rods. After they had been severely flogged, they were thrown into prison, and the jailer was commanded to guard them carefully. Upon receiving such orders, he put them in the inner cell and fastened their feet in the stocks.

About midnight, Paul and Silas were praying and singing hymns to God, and the other prisoners were listening to them. Suddenly, there was such a violent earthquake that the foundations of the prison were shaken. At once all the prison doors flew open, and everyone's chains came loose.

The jailer woke up and, seeing the prison doors open, drew his sword and was about to kill himself because he thought the prisoners had escaped. But Paul shouted, "Don't harm yourself! We are all here!"

The jailer called for lights, rushed in, and fell trembling before Paul and Silas. He then brought them out and asked, "Sirs, what must I do to be saved?"

They replied, "Believe in the Lord Jesus, and you will be saved—you and your household."

Then they spoke the word of the Lord to him and to all the others in his house. At that hour of the night the jailer took them and washed their wounds; then immediately he and all his household were baptized. The jailer brought them into his house and set a meal before them; he was filled with joy because he had come to believe in God—he and his whole household.

The next morning, the magistrates sent their officers to the jailer with the order: "Release those men." The jailer told Paul, "The magistrates have ordered that you and Silas be released. You can leave now. Go in peace."

Paul and Silas's imprisonment in Philippi demonstrates their unwavering faith and commitment to spreading the gospel, even in the face of opposition and suffering. Through their testimony and miraculous deliverance, many, including the jailer and his household, came to believe in Jesus Christ, experiencing salvation and new life.

66. Paul Preaches in Athens

Acts 17:16-34

As Paul waited for his companions in Athens, he was greatly distressed to see the city full of idols. So, he reasoned in the synagogue with both Jews and God-fearing Greeks, as well as in the marketplace day by day with those who happened to be there.

Some of the Epicurean and Stoic philosophers began to debate with him. They said, "What is this babbler trying to say?" Others remarked, "He seems to be advocating foreign gods." They said this because Paul was preaching the good news about Jesus and the resurrection.

Then they took him and brought him to a meeting of the Areopagus, where they said to him, "May we know what this new teaching is that you are presenting? You are bringing some strange ideas to our ears, and we would like to know what they mean."

Paul then stood up in the meeting of the Areopagus and said: "People of Athens! I see that in every way you are very religious. For as I walked around and looked carefully at your objects of worship, I even found an altar with this inscription: to an unknown god. So you are ignorant of the very thing you worship—and this is what I am going to proclaim to you.

"The God who made the world and everything in it is the Lord of heaven and earth and does not live in temples built by human hands. And he is not served by human hands, as if he needed anything. Rather, he himself gives everyone life and breath and everything else.

"From one man he made all the nations, that they should inhabit the whole earth; and he marked out their appointed times in history and the boundaries of their lands. God did this so that they would seek him and perhaps reach out for him and find him, though he is not far from any one of us.

"'For in him we live and move and have our being.' As some of your own poets have said, 'We are his offspring.'

"Therefore since we are God's offspring, we should not think that the divine being is like gold or silver or stone—an image made by human design and skill. In the past, God overlooked such ignorance, but now he commands all people everywhere to repent.

"For he has set a day when he will judge the world with justice by the man he has appointed. He has given proof of this to everyone by raising him from the dead."

When they heard about the resurrection of the dead, some of them sneered, but others said, "We want to hear you again on this subject." At that, Paul left the Council. Some of the people became followers of Paul and believed. Among them was Dionysius, a member of the Areopagus, also a woman named Damaris, and a number of others.

Paul's preaching in Athens showcases his adaptability and boldness in sharing the gospel with diverse audiences. Despite the city's pervasive idolatry and philosophical skepticism, Paul engaged with the Athenians, addressing their spiritual hunger and pointing them to the one true God revealed in Jesus Christ. Though his message was met with mixed reactions, some were receptive and embraced faith in Christ, demonstrating the transformative power of the gospel in the most intellectually and culturally sophisticated contexts.

67. Paul Writes to the Corinthians

1 Corinthians 1:1-9

Paul, called to be an apostle of Christ Jesus by the will of God, and Sosthenes our brother, writes this letter to the church of God in Corinth, to those sanctified in Christ Jesus and called to be his holy people, together with all those everywhere who call on the name of our Lord Jesus Christ—their Lord and ours.

Grace and peace to you from God our Father and the Lord Jesus Christ.

I always thank my God for you because of the grace given you in Christ Jesus. For in him you have been enriched in every way—with all kinds of speech and with all knowledge—God thus confirming our testimony about Christ among you. Therefore you do not lack any spiritual gift as you eagerly wait for our Lord Jesus Christ to be revealed. He will also keep you firm to the end, so that you will be blameless on the day of our Lord Jesus Christ. God is faithful, who has called you into fellowship with his Son, Jesus Christ our Lord.

In his letter to the Corinthians, Paul expresses gratitude for their faithfulness and reminds them of the grace and spiritual gifts they have received through Jesus Christ. He assures them of God's faithfulness and the certainty of Christ's return, encouraging them to remain steadfast in their faith and eagerly anticipate the day of his coming. Paul's words serve as a source of encouragement and reassurance to the Corinthians, emphasizing God's faithfulness and their secure position in Christ.

68. Paul's Shipwreck

Acts 27:13-44

As Paul and his companions set sail from Fair Havens, they encountered strong winds blowing from the northeast called the "northeaster." The ship was caught by the storm and unable to head into the wind, so they gave up and let it be driven along.

After many days of being battered by the storm, with no sun or stars visible for many days and with no hope of being saved, Paul stood up among them and said, "Men, you should have taken my advice not to sail from Crete; then you would have spared yourselves this damage and loss. But now I urge you to keep up your courage, because not one of you will be lost; only the ship will be destroyed. Last night an angel of the God to whom I belong and whom I serve stood beside me and said, 'Do not be afraid, Paul. You must stand trial before Caesar; and God has graciously given you the lives of all who sail with you.' So keep up your courage, men, for I have faith in God that it will happen just as he told me. Nevertheless, we must run aground on some island."

On the fourteenth night, they were still being driven across the Adriatic Sea. About midnight the sailors sensed they were approaching land. They took soundings and found that the water was a hundred and twenty feet deep. A short time later they took soundings again and found it was ninety feet deep. Fearing that they would be dashed against the rocks, they dropped four anchors from the stern and prayed for daylight.

Just before dawn, Paul urged them all to eat. "For the last fourteen days," he said, "you have been in constant suspense and have gone without food—you haven't eaten anything. Now I urge you to take some food. You need it to survive. Not one of you will lose a single hair from his head."

After he said this, he took some bread and gave thanks to God in front of them all. Then he broke it and began to eat. They were all encouraged and ate some food themselves. Altogether there were 276 of us on board.

When they had eaten as much as they wanted, they lightened the ship by throwing the grain into the sea.

When daylight came, they did not recognize the land, but they saw a bay with a sandy beach, where they decided to run the ship aground if they could. Cutting loose the anchors, they left them in the sea and at the same time untied the ropes that held the rudders. Then they hoisted the foresail to the wind and made for the beach. But the ship struck a sandbar and ran aground. The bow stuck fast and would not move, and the stern was broken to pieces by the pounding of the surf.

The soldiers planned to kill the prisoners to prevent any of them from swimming away and escaping. But the centurion wanted to spare Paul's life and kept them from carrying out their plan. He ordered those who could swim to jump overboard first and get to land. The rest were to get there on planks or on other pieces of the ship. In this way everyone reached land safely.

Paul's shipwreck, as described in the book of Acts, is a remarkable account of God's faithfulness and protection amidst adversity. Despite the perilous circumstances, Paul's trust in God's promise of safety and deliverance, as conveyed through an angelic visitation, inspires courage and hope among the crew and passengers. The narrative demonstrates God's sovereign control over nature and his provision for those who belong to him, as Paul's unwavering faith sustains him and ultimately leads to the salvation of all on board.

69. Paul's Letter to the Romans

Romans 1:1-7

Paul, a servant of Christ Jesus, called to be an apostle and set apart for the gospel of God— writes this letter to all in Rome who are loved by God and called to be his holy people:

Grace and peace to you from God our Father and from the Lord Jesus Christ.

First, I thank my God through Jesus Christ for all of you, because your faith is being reported all over the world. God, whom I serve in my spirit in preaching the gospel of his Son, is my witness how constantly I remember you in my prayers at all times; and I pray that now at last by God's will the way may be opened for me to come to you.

I long to see you so that I may impart to you some spiritual gift to make you strong— that is, that you and I may be mutually encouraged by each other's faith. I do not want you to be unaware, brothers and sisters, that I planned many times to come to you (but have been prevented from doing so until now) in order that I might have a harvest among you, just as I have had among the other Gentiles.

I am obligated both to Greeks and non-Greeks, both to the wise and the foolish. That is why I am so eager to preach the gospel also to you who are in Rome.

Paul's letter to the Romans reflects his desire to visit them and share the gospel, affirming their faith and expressing his longing for fellowship with them. His words convey his gratitude for their reputation of faithfulness and his anticipation of mutual encouragement through their shared belief in Jesus Christ. Paul's eagerness to preach the gospel to all, irrespective of their background, underscores his commitment to spreading the message of salvation to the ends of the earth.

70. Paul's Imprisonment in Rome

Acts 28:16-31

When Paul arrived in Rome, the centurion handed him over to the commander of the imperial guard. They allowed Paul to live by himself with a soldier to guard him.

After three days, Paul called together the local Jewish leaders. When they had assembled, Paul said to them: "My brothers, although I have done nothing against our people or against the customs of our ancestors, I was arrested in Jerusalem and handed over to the Romans. They examined me and wanted to release me, because I was not guilty of any crime deserving death. But when the Jews objected, I was compelled to appeal to Caesar—even though I have no charge to bring against my nation. For this reason, I have asked to see you and talk with you. It is because of the hope of Israel that I am bound with this chain."

They replied, "We have not received any letters from Judea concerning you, and none of our people who have come from there has reported or said anything bad about you. But we want to hear what your views are, for we know that people everywhere are talking against this sect."

They arranged to meet Paul on a certain day, and came in even larger numbers to the place where he was staying. He witnessed to them from morning till evening, explaining about the kingdom of God, and from the Law of Moses and from the Prophets he tried to persuade them about Jesus. Some were convinced by what he said, but others would not believe. They disagreed among themselves and began to leave after Paul had made this final statement: "The Holy Spirit spoke the truth to your ancestors when he said through Isaiah the prophet:

"'Go to this people and say,
"You will be ever hearing but never understanding;
you will be ever seeing but never perceiving."
For this people's heart has become calloused;
they hardly hear with their ears,
and they have closed their eyes.
Otherwise they might see with their eyes,
hear with their ears,
understand with their hearts
and turn, and I would heal them.'

"Therefore I want you to know that God's salvation has been sent to the Gentiles, and they will listen!"

For two whole years Paul stayed there in his own rented house and welcomed all who came to see him. He proclaimed the kingdom of God and taught about the Lord Jesus Christ—with all boldness and without hindrance.

Paul's imprisonment in Rome marks a pivotal moment in his ministry, as he continues to proclaim the gospel despite being under house arrest. Even while confined, Paul seizes every opportunity to share the message of Jesus Christ with both Jews and Gentiles, testifying to the kingdom of God and persuading others to believe. Despite facing opposition and rejection, Paul remains steadfast in his commitment to spreading the good news, demonstrating unwavering faith and determination until the end of his imprisonment.

71. Peter Preaches to the Gentiles

Acts 10:34-48

Then Peter began to speak: "I now realize how true it is that God does not show favoritism but accepts from every nation the one who fears him and does what is right. You know the message God sent to the people of Israel, announcing the good news of peace through Jesus Christ, who is Lord of all. You know what has happened throughout the province of Judea, beginning in Galilee after the baptism that John preached—how God anointed Jesus of Nazareth with the Holy Spirit and power, and how he went around doing good and healing all who were under the power of the devil because God was with him.

"We are witnesses of everything he did in the country of the Jews and in Jerusalem. They killed him by hanging him on a cross, but God raised him from the dead on the third day and caused him to be seen. He was not seen by all the people, but by witnesses whom God had already chosen—by us who ate and drank with him after he rose from the dead. He commanded us to preach to the people and to testify that he is the one whom God appointed as judge of the living and the dead. All the prophets testify about him that everyone who believes in him receives forgiveness of sins through his name."

While Peter was still speaking these words, the Holy Spirit came on all who heard the message. The circumcised believers who had come with Peter were astonished that the gift of the Holy Spirit had been poured out even on Gentiles. For they heard them speaking in tongues and praising God.

Then Peter said, "Surely no one can stand in the way of their being baptized with water. They have received the Holy Spirit just as we have." So he ordered that they be baptized in the name of Jesus Christ. Then they asked Peter to stay with them for a few days.

Peter's preaching to the Gentiles marks a pivotal moment in the early Christian church, as he recognizes God's acceptance of Gentiles into the community of believers. His message emphasizes the universal nature of the gospel, proclaiming Jesus Christ as Lord and Savior for all people, regardless of their nationality or background. The outpouring of the Holy Spirit on the Gentile listeners validates their inclusion in the body of

Christ, prompting Peter to baptize them in the name of Jesus. This event highlights the transformative power of the gospel and God's impartial love for all humanity.

72. James' Letter to the Twelve Tribes

James 1:1-8

James, a servant of God and of the Lord Jesus Christ, writes this letter to the twelve tribes scattered among the nations:

Greetings to you all!

Consider it pure joy, my brothers and sisters, whenever you face trials of many kinds because you know that the testing of your faith produces perseverance. Let perseverance finish its work so that you may be mature and complete, not lacking anything. If any of you lacks wisdom, you should ask God, who gives generously to all without finding fault, and it will be given to you. But when you ask, you must believe and not doubt, because the one who doubts is like a wave of the sea, blown and tossed by the wind. That person should not expect to receive anything from the Lord. Such a person is double-minded and unstable in all they do.

In his letter addressed to the twelve tribes, James encourages believers to find joy amidst trials, recognizing them as opportunities for spiritual growth. He emphasizes the importance of perseverance, trusting that trials refine faith and lead to maturity. James highlights the accessibility of God's wisdom, urging readers to seek it with unwavering faith. He warns against doubt, likening it to a wavering wave that undermines one's ability to receive from God. James emphasizes the necessity of single-minded devotion to God, as double-mindedness leads to instability in all aspects of life. Through his letter, James offers timeless wisdom and practical guidance to believers, reminding them of God's faithfulness and provision in every circumstance.

73. Revelations

Revelation 1:1-3; 22:18-19

The book of Revelation, written by the apostle John, begins with a revelation from Jesus Christ about events that will soon take place. It is a prophetic vision given to John by an angel, containing the word of God and the testimony of Jesus Christ. The book is intended to be read and heard by believers, as it offers blessings to those who take its words to heart.

Throughout Revelation, John records vivid imagery and symbolic language depicting the ultimate victory of Christ over evil, the establishment of God's kingdom, and the final judgment. The book portrays scenes of heavenly worship, the unveiling of God's plan for redemption, and the defeat of Satan and his forces.

Revelation also includes messages to seven churches, encouraging believers to remain faithful amidst persecution and to repent of their sins. It warns of impending judgment for those who reject God's grace and persist in wickedness.

In the concluding verses, John emphasizes the importance of preserving the integrity of the prophecy contained in Revelation, warning against adding or subtracting from its words under penalty of divine judgment.

Overall, the book of Revelation serves as a powerful reminder of God's sovereignty, the triumph of good over evil, and the hope of eternal life for those who trust in Jesus Christ.

74. The Healing of the Blind Man

John 9:1-12

In the town, there was a man who had been blind since birth. People knew him well; he was often seen sitting by the roadside, begging for alms. One day, as Jesus and his disciples walked by, they noticed the blind man.

Curious, the disciples asked Jesus, "Teacher, why was this man born blind? Did he sin, or did his parents sin?"

Jesus replied, "Neither this man nor his parents sinned. This happened so that the works of God might be displayed in him. While it is daytime, we must do the works of him who sent me. Night is coming when no one can work. While I am in the world, I am the light of the world."

After saying this, Jesus spat on the ground, made mud with the saliva, and spread it on the blind man's eyes. Then he told him, "Go, wash in the Pool of Siloam."

The blind man did as Jesus commanded, and as he washed, his sight was restored. Overjoyed, he returned home, seeing the world for the first time.

His neighbors and those who had seen him begging were amazed. Some said, "Isn't this the man who used to sit and beg?" Others said, "No, he only looks like him."

But the man insisted, "I am the one!"

They asked him, "How were your eyes opened?"

He answered, "The man they call Jesus made mud and put it on my eyes. Then he told me to go and wash. So I went and washed, and then I could see."

Puzzled, they inquired further, "Where is this man?"

The man replied, "I do not know."

Tthis story teaches us about Jesus' compassion, the purpose in suffering, the importance of faith and obedience, and the impact of witnessing God's miraculous works in our lives. It encourages us to trust in Jesus, obey his commands, and share our experiences of his grace and power with others.

75. The Compassion of Jesus

John 8:1-11

In the temple courtyard, Jesus was teaching a crowd of people who had gathered to listen to him. Suddenly, the religious leaders brought in a woman caught in the act of adultery. They stood her in front of everyone and said to Jesus, "Teacher, this woman was caught in the act of adultery. The law of Moses commands us to stone such women. What do you say?"

But Jesus stooped down and started writing on the ground with his finger, ignoring their question. When they kept demanding an answer, Jesus stood up and said to them, "Let any one of you who is without sin be the first to throw a stone at her."

Then he stooped down and continued writing on the ground. One by one, starting with the oldest, the accusers left until only Jesus and the woman remained.

Jesus looked up and asked her, "Woman, where are they? Has no one condemned you?"

"No one, sir," she replied.

"Then neither do I condemn you," Jesus declared. "Go now and leave your life of sin."

This encounter reveals Jesus's compassion and wisdom. He doesn't condone the woman's sin but offers her forgiveness and a chance to start anew. Instead of condemning her, he challenges her accusers to examine their own hearts. Jesus's response teaches us about the importance of forgiveness, compassion, and humility. He shows us that true justice is balanced with mercy and that everyone, regardless of their past mistakes, has the opportunity to experience grace and transformation.

The Good Samaritan
Luke 10:25-37

A man approached Jesus and asked, "Teacher, what must I do to inherit eternal life?"

Jesus replied, "What is written in the Law? How do you understand it?"

The man answered, "Love the Lord your God with all your heart, soul, strength, and mind, and love your neighbor as yourself."

"You have answered correctly," Jesus said. "Do this, and you will live."

But the man wanted to justify himself, so he asked, "And who is my neighbor?"

In response, Jesus told a story:

"A man was traveling from Jerusalem to Jericho when he fell into the hands of robbers. They stripped him, beat him, and left him half dead. A priest happened to be going down the same road, but when he saw the injured man, he passed by on the other side. Then a Levite came, but he too walked by without helping.

But a Samaritan, as he traveled, came where the man was; and when he saw him, he took pity on him. He went to him, bandaged his wounds, poured oil and wine on them, and took him to an inn. The next day, he gave money to the innkeeper and said, 'Look after him. When I return, I will reimburse you for any extra expense.'

Jesus then asked, "Which of these three do you think was a neighbor to the man who fell into the hands of robbers?"

The man replied, "The one who showed him mercy."

Jesus told him, "Go and do likewise."

76. The Prodigal Son

Luke 15:11-32

A man had two sons. The younger son said to his father, "Father, give me my share of the estate." So the father divided his property between his two sons.

Not long after that, the younger son gathered all he had and went to a distant country. There he squandered his wealth in wild living. After he had spent everything, a severe famine hit the land, and he began to be in need. So he hired himself out to a citizen of that country, who sent him to his fields to feed pigs. He longed to fill his stomach with the pods that the pigs were eating, but no one gave him anything.

When he came to his senses, he said, "How many of my father's hired servants have food to spare, and here I am starving to death! I will go back to my father and say to him: Father, I have sinned against heaven and against you. I am no longer worthy to be called your son; make me like one of your hired servants."

So he got up and went to his father. But while he was still a long way off, his father saw him and was filled with compassion for him; he ran to his son, threw his arms around him and kissed him.

The son said to him, "Father, I have sinned against heaven and against you. I am no longer worthy to be called your son."

But the father said to his servants, "Quick! Bring the best robe and put it on him. Put a ring on his finger and sandals on his feet. Bring the fattened calf and kill it. Let's have a feast and celebrate. For this son of mine was dead and is alive again; he was lost and is found." So they began to celebrate.

Meanwhile, the older son was in the field. When he came near the house, he heard music and dancing. So he called one of the servants and asked him what was going on. "Your brother has come," he replied, "and your father has killed the fattened calf because he has him back safe and sound."

The older brother became angry and refused to go in. So his father went out and pleaded with him. But he answered his father, "Look! All these years I've been slaving for you and never disobeyed your orders. Yet you never gave me even a young goat so I could celebrate with my friends. But when this son of yours who has squandered your property with prostitutes comes home, you kill the fattened calf for him!"

"My son," the father said, "you are always with me, and everything I have is yours. But we had to celebrate and be glad, because this brother of yours was dead and is alive again; he was lost and is found."

77. The Pharisee and the Tax Collector

Luke 18:9-14

Jesus told a story to some people who thought they were better than others. He said:

"Two men went to the temple to pray. One was a Pharisee, a religious leader who thought highly of himself. The other was a tax collector, a man despised by many because of his profession.

The Pharisee stood by himself and prayed, 'God, I thank you that I am not like other people—robbers, evildoers, adulterers—or even like this tax collector. I fast twice a week and give a tenth of all I get.'

But the tax collector stood at a distance. He would not even look up to heaven, but beat his breast and said, 'God, have mercy on me, a sinner.'

Jesus said, "I tell you that this tax collector, rather than the Pharisee, went home justified before God. For all those who exalt themselves will be humbled, and those who humble themselves will be exalted."

This story teaches us about humility and self-righteousness. The Pharisee, proud of his religious achievements, looked down on others and boasted about his own righteousness. In contrast, the tax collector recognized his sinfulness and pleaded for God's mercy with a humble heart.

Jesus's message is clear: God values humility over pride. Those who recognize their need for mercy and approach God with humility will be justified in his sight. We are reminded to avoid self-righteousness and instead acknowledge our dependence on God's grace for forgiveness and salvation.

78. The Rich Man and Lazarus

Luke 16:19-31

Jesus told a story about a rich man and a beggar named Lazarus:

There was a rich man who dressed in fine clothes and feasted luxuriously every day. At his gate was a beggar named Lazarus, covered with sores and longing to eat scraps from the rich man's table. Even the dogs came and licked Lazarus' sores.

One day, Lazarus died and was carried by the angels to Abraham's side in heaven. The rich man also died and was buried. In Hades, where he was in torment, he looked up and saw Abraham far away, with Lazarus by his side.

The rich man called out, "Father Abraham, have pity on me and send Lazarus to dip the tip of his finger in water and cool my tongue, because I am in agony in this fire."

But Abraham replied, "Son, remember that in your lifetime you received your good things, while Lazarus received bad things. Now he is comforted here, and you are in agony. Besides, there is a great chasm between us and you, so that those who want to go from here to you cannot, nor can anyone cross over from there to us."

The rich man pleaded, "Then I beg you, father, send Lazarus to my family, for I have five brothers. Let him warn them so that they will not also come to this place of torment."

Abraham replied, "They have Moses and the Prophets; let them listen to them."

"No, father Abraham," the rich man said, "but if someone from the dead goes to them, they will repent."

Abraham responded, "If they do not listen to Moses and the Prophets, they will not be convinced even if someone rises from the dead."

This reminds us that wealth and status in this world do not guarantee favor with God, and that true value lies in showing kindness and mercy to those in need. it emphasizes the need for repentance and faith in God, as well as the urgency of sharing the message of salvation with others.

79. The Lost Sheep

Luke 15:3-7

Jesus shared a story about a shepherd who had a flock of one hundred sheep. One day, he realized that one of his sheep was missing. He left the ninety-nine sheep in the open field and went in search of the lost one.

The shepherd searched far and wide, calling out for the lost sheep. He climbed hills, crossed valleys, and navigated through thickets until finally, he found the lost sheep stuck in a thorn bush.

With great relief, the shepherd gently lifted the lost sheep from the thorns and placed it on his shoulders. He carried it back to the flock, rejoicing all the way. When he arrived home, he called together his friends and neighbors and said, "Rejoice with me! I have found my lost sheep!"

In the same way, Jesus explained, there is more joy in heaven over one sinner who repents than over ninety-nine righteous people who do not need to repent.

This story illustrates the depth of God's love and his relentless pursuit of those who are lost. Like the shepherd who tirelessly searched for his lost sheep, God actively seeks out every lost soul, longing for them to return to him.

As believers, we are called to share in God's heart for the lost, to actively reach out and bring them back into the fold. Just as the shepherd rejoiced over finding his lost sheep, so too does God rejoice when a lost soul is found and returns to him.

80. The Lost Coin

Luke 15:8-10

In a small village, there lived a woman who had ten silver coins. One day, as she was tidying up her home, she realized that one of her coins was missing. Distressed, she lit a lamp and began to search carefully, sweeping every corner of the house.

After much searching, she finally found the lost coin hidden under a pile of dust in a dark corner. Overjoyed, she called her friends and neighbors together, saying, "Rejoice with me! I have found my lost coin!"

In the same way, Jesus explained, there is joy in the presence of the angels of God over one sinner who repents.

This simple yet profound story illustrates God's relentless pursuit of every lost soul. The woman's diligent search for her lost coin reflects God's unwavering commitment to seek out and restore those who are lost.

Like the lost coin, each person holds great value in God's eyes. He desires that none should perish but that all should come to repentance. Therefore, he actively searches for those who are lost, longing to bring them back into his loving embrace.

We are called to share in God's heart for the lost, to engage in seeking and rescuing those who have strayed away from him. Just as the woman rejoiced over finding her lost coin, so too does God rejoice when a lost soul is found and returns to him. And in that moment, there is great celebration in heaven over the repentance of one sinner.

81. The Lost Son

Luke 15:11-32

There was once a man who had two sons. The younger son said to his father, "Father, give me my share of the estate." So the father divided his property between his two sons.

Not long after, the younger son gathered all he had and journeyed to a distant country, where he squandered his wealth in reckless living. When he had spent everything, a severe famine struck that land, and he found himself in desperate need.

In his distress, the young man hired himself out to a citizen of that country, who sent him into his fields to feed pigs. He was so hungry that he longed to eat the pods the pigs were eating, but no one gave him anything.

Finally, he came to his senses and said, "How many of my father's hired servants have food to spare, and here I am starving to death! I will go back to my father and say to him: 'Father, I have sinned against heaven and against you. I am no longer worthy to be called your son; make me like one of your hired servants.'"

So he set off and went to his father. But while he was still a long way off, his father saw him and was filled with compassion. He ran to his son, threw his arms around him, and kissed him.

The son said to him, "Father, I have sinned against heaven and against you. I am no longer worthy to be called your son."

But the father said to his servants, "Quick! Bring the best robe and put it on him. Put a ring on his finger and sandals on his feet. Bring the fattened calf and kill it. Let's have a feast and celebrate. For this son of mine was dead and is alive again; he was lost and is found."

And so the celebration began for the return of the lost son.

82. The Parable of the Sower

Matthew 13:3-9

Jesus told a story to a large crowd gathered by the lakeside:

"A farmer went out to sow his seed. As he scattered the seed, some fell along the path, and the birds came and ate it up. Some fell on rocky places, where it did not have much soil. It sprang up quickly because the soil was shallow. But when the sun came up, the plants were scorched, and they withered because they had no root. Other seed fell among thorns, which grew up and choked the plants. Still, other seed fell on good soil, where it produced a crop—a hundred, sixty, or thirty times what was sown. Whoever has ears, let them hear."

Later, when Jesus was alone with his disciples, they asked him about the meaning of the parable.

Jesus explained, "The seed represents the message about the kingdom of God. The soil represents different types of hearts. The seed that fell along the path represents those who hear the word of God but do not understand it. The evil one comes and snatches away what was sown in their hearts. The seed on rocky ground represents those who hear the word and receive it with joy, but they have no root and fall away when troubles or persecution come because of the word. The seed among thorns represents those who hear the word, but the worries of this life and the deceitfulness of wealth choke the word, making it unfruitful. The seed on good soil represents those who hear the word, understand it, and produce a crop—a hundred, sixty, or thirty times what was sown."

Jesus concluded, "Let those with ears, listen and understand."

83. The Parable of the Mustard Seed

Matthew 13:31-32

Jesus shared another parable with the crowd:

"The kingdom of heaven is like a mustard seed that a man planted in his field. Though it is the smallest of all seeds, yet when it grows, it is the largest of garden plants and becomes a tree, so that the birds come and perch in its branches."

Jesus used this simple story to illustrate the incredible growth and impact of the kingdom of heaven. Despite starting as something small and seemingly insignificant, like a tiny mustard seed, the kingdom of heaven grows into something great and expansive, providing shelter and sustenance for many.

Just as a mustard seed grows into a large tree, so too does the kingdom of heaven expand and flourish in the hearts of people. It starts small, perhaps with a single act of kindness or a small community of believers, but it has the potential to grow and spread far and wide, impacting the lives of many.

This parable encourages us to have faith in the power and potential of God's kingdom. Even when things seem small or insignificant, God can work miracles and bring about incredible growth and transformation. We are reminded that God's kingdom is not limited by human understanding or expectations but is expansive and inclusive, inviting all to find refuge and hope in its branches.

84. The Parable of the Wheat and the Tares

Matthew 13:24-30

Jesus told a story to the crowd:

"The kingdom of heaven is like a man who sowed good seed in his field. But while everyone was sleeping, his enemy came and sowed weeds among the wheat and went away. When the wheat sprouted and formed heads, the weeds also appeared.

The owner's servants came to him and asked, 'Sir, didn't you sow good seed in your field? Where then did the weeds come from?'

'An enemy did this,' he replied.

The servants asked him, 'Do you want us to go and pull them up?'

'No,' he answered, 'because while you are pulling the weeds, you may uproot the wheat with them. Let both grow together until the harvest. At that time, I will tell the harvesters: First, collect the weeds and tie them in bundles to be burned; then gather the wheat and bring it into my barn.'"

Jesus later explained the meaning of the parable to his disciples:

"The one who sowed the good seed is the Son of Man, and the field is the world. The good seed stands for the people of the kingdom, while the weeds are the people of the evil one. The enemy who sows them is the devil. The harvest is the end of the age, and the harvesters are angels.

Just as the weeds are pulled up and burned in the fire, so it will be at the end of the age. The Son of Man will send out his angels, and they will weed out of his kingdom everything that causes sin and all who do evil. They will throw them into the blazing furnace, where there will be weeping and gnashing of teeth. Then the righteous will shine like the sun in the kingdom of their Father."

85. The Parable of the Good Shepherd

John 10:11-18

Jesus shared a story with the people:

"I am the good shepherd. The good shepherd lays down his life for the sheep. The hired hand is not the shepherd and does not own the sheep. So when he sees the wolf coming, he abandons the sheep and runs away. Then the wolf attacks the flock and scatters it. The man runs away because he is a hired hand and cares nothing for the sheep.

But I am the good shepherd; I know my sheep and my sheep know me—just as the Father knows me and I know the Father—and I lay down my life for the sheep. I have other sheep that are not of this sheep pen. I must bring them also. They too will listen to my voice, and there shall be one flock and one shepherd. The reason my Father loves me is that I lay down my life—only to take it up again. No one takes it from me, but I lay it down of my own accord. I have authority to lay it down and authority to take it up again. This command I received from my Father."

Jesus used the analogy of a shepherd caring for his sheep to illustrate his deep love and sacrificial care for his followers. He emphasized his willingness to lay down his life for them, contrasting it with the actions of a hired hand who abandons the sheep in times of danger. Jesus assured his listeners that he knows each of his sheep intimately and is willing to bring all who believe in him into his fold, ensuring their safety and unity under his loving care.

86. The Parable of the Vineyard Workers

Matthew 20:1-16

Jesus told a story to his disciples:

"The kingdom of heaven is like a landowner who went out early in the morning to hire workers for his vineyard. He agreed to pay them a denarius for the day's work and sent them into his vineyard.

About nine in the morning, he went out and saw others standing in the marketplace doing nothing. He told them, 'You also go and work in my vineyard, and I will pay you whatever is right.' So they went.

At noon and again at three in the afternoon, he did the same thing. About five in the afternoon, he went out and found still others standing around. He asked them, 'Why have you been standing here all day long doing nothing?'

'Because no one has hired us,' they answered.

He said to them, 'You also go and work in my vineyard.'

When evening came, the owner of the vineyard said to his foreman, 'Call the workers and pay them their wages, beginning with the last ones hired and going on to the first.'

The workers who were hired about five in the afternoon came and each received a denarius. So when those came who were hired first, they expected to receive more. But each one of them also received a denarius.

When they received it, they began to grumble against the landowner. 'These who were hired last worked only one hour,' they said, 'and you have made them equal to us who have borne the burden of the work and the heat of the day.'

But he answered one of them, 'I am not being unfair to you, friend. Didn't you agree to work for a denarius? Take your pay and go. I want to give the one who was hired last the same as I gave you. Don't I have the right to do what I want with my own money? Or are you envious because I am generous?'"

Jesus concluded, "So the last will be first, and the first will be last."

87. The Parable of the Talents

Matthew 25:14-30

Jesus shared a story with his disciples:

"The kingdom of heaven is like a man going on a journey, who called his servants and entrusted his wealth to them. To one he gave five bags of gold, to another two bags, and to another one bag, each according to his ability. Then he went on his journey.

The man who had received five bags of gold went at once and put his money to work and gained five bags more. So also, the one with two bags of gold gained two more. But the man who had received one bag went off, dug a hole in the ground, and hid his master's money.

After a long time, the master of those servants returned and settled accounts with them. The man who had received five bags of gold brought the other five. 'Master,' he said, 'you entrusted me with five bags of gold. See, I have gained five more.'

His master replied, 'Well done, good and faithful servant! You have been faithful with a few things; I will put you in charge of many things. Come and share your master's happiness!'

The man with two bags of gold also came. 'Master,' he said, 'you entrusted me with two bags of gold; see, I have gained two more.'

His master replied, 'Well done, good and faithful servant! You have been faithful with a few things; I will put you in charge of many things. Come and share your master's happiness!'

Then the man who had received one bag of gold came. 'Master,' he said, 'I knew that you are a hard man, harvesting where you have not sown and gathering where you have not scattered seed. So I was afraid and went out and hid your gold in the ground. See, here is what belongs to you.'

His master replied, 'You wicked, lazy servant! So you knew that I harvest where I have not sown and gather where I have not scattered seed? Well then, you should have put my money on deposit with the bankers, so that when I returned I would have received it back with interest.

'Take the bag of gold from him and give it to the one who has ten bags. For whoever has will be given more, and they will have an abundance. Whoever does not have, even what they have will be taken from them. And throw that worthless servant outside, into the darkness, where there will be weeping and gnashing of teeth.'"

Jesus concluded, "For whoever has will be given more, and they will have an abundance. Whoever does not have, even what they have will be taken from them."

88. The Parable of the Wise and Foolish Builders

Matthew 7:24-27

Jesus told his disciples a story:

"Everyone who hears these words of mine and puts them into practice is like a wise man who built his house on the rock. The rain came down, the streams rose, and the winds blew and beat against that house; yet it did not fall, because it had its foundation on the rock.

"But everyone who hears these words of mine and does not put them into practice is like a foolish man who built his house on sand. The rain came down, the streams rose, and the winds blew and beat against that house, and it fell with a great crash."

Jesus used this simple story to teach his disciples about the importance of not only hearing his teachings but also putting them into practice. He compared those who obeyed his words to a wise builder who laid a solid foundation for his house on a rock. When the storms came, the house stood firm because of its strong foundation.

On the other hand, those who heard Jesus' words but did not follow them were like a foolish builder who built his house on sand. When the storms came, the house collapsed because it lacked a sturdy foundation.

This parable reminds us that true wisdom comes from obeying Jesus' teachings and living them out in our lives. It's not enough to simply hear his words; we must also act upon them. By doing so, we establish a firm foundation for our lives that can withstand the trials and challenges that come our way.

89. The Parable of the Rich Fool

Luke 12:16-21

Jesus shared a parable with the crowd:

"The ground of a certain rich man yielded an abundant harvest. He thought to himself, 'What shall I do? I have no place to store my crops.'

"Then he said, 'This is what I'll do. I will tear down my barns and build bigger ones, and there I will store my surplus grain. And I'll say to myself, "You have plenty of grain laid up for many years. Take life easy; eat, drink and be merry."'

"But God said to him, 'You fool! This very night your life will be demanded from you. Then who will get what you have prepared for yourself?'

"This is how it will be with whoever stores up things for themselves but is not rich toward God."

In this parable, Jesus warned against the dangers of greed and selfishness. The rich man in the story was focused solely on his own wealth and comfort, with no consideration for others or for God. He hoarded his abundance of crops, planning to live a life of leisure and indulgence. However, his plans were cut short when God called him to account for his life.

This parable serves as a reminder to prioritize spiritual wealth over material possessions. True richness comes from being generous and faithful toward God, rather than accumulating earthly wealth for selfish gain. Jesus encourages us to seek first the kingdom of God and his righteousness, trusting that all our needs will be provided for, and that our true treasure is found in a relationship with God, rather than in earthly riches.

90. The Parable of The Persistent Widow

Luke 18:1-8

Jesus told his disciples a story:

"There was once a judge in a certain town who neither feared God nor cared about people. There was also a widow in that town who kept coming to him with the plea, 'Grant me justice against my adversary.'

"For some time he refused. But finally he said to himself, 'Even though I don't fear God or care what people think, yet because this widow keeps bothering me, I will see that she gets justice, so that she won't eventually come and attack me!'"

Then the Lord said, "Listen to what the unjust judge says. And will not God bring about justice for his chosen ones, who cry out to him day and night? Will he keep putting them off? I tell you, he will see that they get justice, and quickly. However, when the Son of Man comes, will he find faith on the earth?"

In this parable, Jesus taught about the importance of persistent prayer. The widow in the story persisted in seeking justice from the unjust judge, and eventually, her persistence paid off. Jesus used this parable to encourage his followers to pray continually and not lose heart. He assured them that God, who is just and loving, will hear and answer their prayers in his perfect timing. Thus, he urged them to remain faithful and persistent in their prayers, trusting in God's faithfulness to fulfill his promises.

91. The Parable of the Pharisee and the Publican

Luke 18:9-14

Jesus told a story to some who were confident of their own righteousness and looked down on everyone else:

"Two men went up to the temple to pray, one a Pharisee and the other a tax collector. The Pharisee stood by himself and prayed: 'God, I thank you that I am not like other people—robbers, evildoers, adulterers—or even like this tax collector. I fast twice a week and give a tenth of all I get.'

"But the tax collector stood at a distance. He would not even look up to heaven, but beat his breast and said, 'God, have mercy on me, a sinner.'

"I tell you that this man, rather than the other, went home justified before God. For all those who exalt themselves will be humbled, and those who humble themselves will be exalted."

In this parable, Jesus contrasts the attitudes of the Pharisee and the tax collector in prayer. The Pharisee, proud of his own righteousness, boasted about his religious observances and looked down on others. In contrast, the tax collector recognized his own sinfulness and humbly sought God's mercy.

Jesus used this parable to teach about the importance of humility and sincerity in prayer. He emphasized that it is not outward displays of religious piety that please God, but rather a humble and repentant heart. Those who exalt themselves will be humbled, but those who humble themselves before God will be exalted in his sight.

92. The Parable of the Wedding Feast

Matthew 22:1-14

Jesus shared another parable with the crowd:

"The kingdom of heaven is like a king who prepared a wedding banquet for his son. He sent his servants to those who had been invited to the banquet to tell them to come, but they refused to come.

"Then he sent some more servants and said, 'Tell those who have been invited that I have prepared my dinner: My oxen and fattened cattle have been butchered, and everything is ready. Come to the wedding banquet.'

"But they paid no attention and went off—one to his field, another to his business. The rest seized his servants, mistreated them, and killed them. The king was enraged. He sent his army and destroyed those murderers and burned their city.

"Then he said to his servants, 'The wedding banquet is ready, but those I invited did not deserve to come. So go to the street corners and invite to the banquet anyone you find.' So the servants went out into the streets and gathered all the people they could find, the bad as well as the good, and the wedding hall was filled with guests.

"But when the king came in to see the guests, he noticed a man there who was not wearing wedding clothes. He asked, 'How did you get in here without wedding clothes, friend?' The man was speechless.

"Then the king told the attendants, 'Tie him hand and foot, and throw him outside, into the darkness, where there will be weeping and gnashing of teeth.'

"For many are invited, but few are chosen."

In this parable, Jesus illustrates the invitation to the kingdom of heaven as a wedding feast. The initial guests, who represent the religious leaders of the time, rejected the invitation, so the king extended it to others, symbolizing the invitation to all people, both good and bad. However, the parable also emphasizes the importance of responding to God's invitation with sincerity and proper attire, symbolizing righteousness.

93. The Parable of the Friend at Midnight

Luke 11:5-8

Jesus told his disciples a story:

"Suppose you have a friend, and you go to him at midnight and say, 'Friend, lend me three loaves of bread; a friend of mine on a journey has come to me, and I have no food to offer him.' And suppose the one inside answers, 'Don't bother me. The door is already locked, and my children and I are in bed. I can't get up and give you anything.'

"I tell you, even though he will not get up and give you the bread because of friendship, yet because of your shameless audacity he will surely get up and give you as much as you need."

In this parable, Jesus illustrates the importance of persistence in prayer. The man goes to his friend's house at midnight seeking bread to offer to his unexpected guest. Despite his friend's initial reluctance due to inconvenience, he eventually responds to the man's persistent request and provides him with what he needs.

Jesus uses this parable to encourage his disciples to persevere in prayer, even when it seems that God is not answering immediately. He assures them that God, who is loving and generous, will respond to their prayers, especially when they approach Him with persistence and faith.

This parable teaches us the value of persistence in prayer and reminds us to trust in God's faithfulness to answer our prayers according to His will and timing. It encourages us to continue seeking God earnestly and to trust in His provision and care for our needs.

94. The Parable of the Unjust Steward

Luke 16:1-13

Jesus told his disciples a story:

There was a rich man whose manager was accused of wasting his possessions. So he called him in and asked him, 'What is this I hear about you? Give an account of your management, because you cannot be manager any longer.'

The manager said to himself, 'What shall I do now? My master is taking away my job. I'm not strong enough to dig, and I'm ashamed to beg— I know what I'll do so that, when I lose my job here, people will welcome me into their houses.'

So he called in each one of his master's debtors. He asked the first, 'How much do you owe my master?'

'Nine hundred gallons of olive oil,' he replied.

The manager told him, 'Take your bill, sit down quickly, and make it four hundred and fifty.'

Then he asked the second, 'And how much do you owe?'

'A thousand bushels of wheat,' he replied.

He told him, 'Take your bill and make it eight hundred.'

The master commended the dishonest manager because he had acted shrewdly. For the people of this world are more shrewd in dealing with their own kind than are the people of the light. I tell you, use worldly wealth to gain friends for yourselves, so that when it is gone, you will be welcomed into eternal dwellings.

In this parable, Jesus uses the example of an unjust steward who, facing dismissal, uses his master's resources to secure his future. Jesus commends the steward's shrewdness but also emphasizes the importance of using worldly wealth wisely and for eternal purposes. He teaches that while worldly wealth is temporary, using it to bless others and further God's kingdom yields eternal rewards.

95. The Parable of the Great Banquet

Luke 14:15-24

Jesus told a story to the guests at a dinner:

"One day, a man prepared a great banquet and invited many guests. When the banquet was ready, he sent his servant to tell those who had been invited, 'Come, for everything is now ready.'

"But they all alike began to make excuses. The first said, 'I have just bought a field, and I must go and see it. Please excuse me.'

"Another said, 'I have just bought five yoke of oxen, and I'm on my way to try them out. Please excuse me.'

"Still, another said, 'I just got married, so I can't come.'

"The servant returned and reported this to his master. Then the owner of the house became angry and ordered his servant, 'Go out quickly into the streets and alleys of the town and bring in the poor, the crippled, the blind and the lame.'

"'Sir,' the servant said, 'what you ordered has been done, but there is still room.'

"Then the master told his servant, 'Go out to the roads and country lanes and compel them to come in, so that my house will be full. I tell you, not one of those who were invited will get a taste of my banquet.'"

In this parable, Jesus illustrates the kingdom of heaven as a great banquet to which many are invited. However, those who were initially invited—representing the religious leaders of the time—rejected the invitation due to their preoccupations and excuses. Instead, the invitation was extended to others, including the poor, the crippled, the blind, and the lame, symbolizing all people, regardless of their status or background. Jesus emphasizes that those who respond to God's invitation with faith will be part of His kingdom, while those who reject it will miss out on the blessings of eternal life.

96. The Parable of the Fig Tree

Matthew 24:32-35

Jesus shared a parable with his disciples:

"Learn a lesson from the fig tree. When its branches become green and soft and new leaves appear, you know summer is near. In the same way, when you see all these things happening, you will know that the time is near, ready to happen. I tell you the truth, all these things will happen while some of the people of this time are still living. The whole world, earth, and sky will be destroyed, but the words I have said will never be destroyed."

In this parable, Jesus uses the fig tree as an illustration of recognizing signs of the times. Just as the appearance of leaves on the fig tree indicates the approach of summer, the signs Jesus described, such as wars, famines, and earthquakes, signal the nearness of His return and the end of the age.

Jesus emphasizes the certainty of His words, assuring His disciples that despite the destruction of the world,

His teachings will endure forever. He urges them to be vigilant and discerning, paying attention to the signs of the times and remaining faithful to His teachings.

This parable serves as a reminder for believers to stay alert and prepared for the coming of the Lord. It encourages them to live with hope and expectancy, knowing that God's promises will be fulfilled and His kingdom will come.

97. The Parable of the Hidden Treasure

Matthew 13:44

Jesus told a story to his followers:

"The kingdom of heaven is like a treasure hidden in a field. One day, a man found the treasure hidden in the field. He was so happy that he went and sold everything he had to buy that field."

In this parable, Jesus compares the kingdom of heaven to a valuable treasure hidden in a field. Just as the man found the treasure and recognized its worth, those who discover the kingdom of heaven understand its priceless value.

The man's reaction to finding the treasure illustrates the response of someone who truly grasps the significance of the kingdom. He is willing to sacrifice everything he owns to obtain it. Similarly, when individuals recognize the worth of God's kingdom, they are willing to give up everything—worldly possessions, ambitions, and desires—to be a part of it.

This parable teaches us about the incomparable value of the kingdom of heaven. It challenges us to prioritize seeking God's kingdom above all else and to be willing to make whatever sacrifices are necessary to obtain it. It also emphasizes the joy and fulfillment that come from knowing and belonging to God's kingdom. Ultimately, the parable encourages us to seek first the kingdom of God, trusting that everything else will fall into place according to His will.

98. The Parable of the Pearl of Great Price

Matthew 13:45-46

Jesus shared another parable with the crowd:

"The kingdom of heaven is like a merchant looking for fine pearls. One day, he found one very precious pearl. He went and sold everything he owned to buy it."

In this parable, Jesus illustrates the value of the kingdom of heaven by comparing it to a precious pearl. Just as the merchant recognized the worth of the pearl and was willing to sacrifice everything to obtain it, those who understand the value of the kingdom of heaven are willing to give up everything to possess it.

The merchant's actions demonstrate the single-minded pursuit of something of great value. He willingly sells all his possessions to acquire the priceless pearl, indicating the supreme importance he places on obtaining it. Similarly, when individuals grasp the significance of the kingdom of heaven, they are willing to relinquish all worldly attachments and ambitions to obtain the eternal blessings it offers.

This parable teaches us about the incomparable worth of the kingdom of heaven and the radical commitment required to obtain it. It challenges us to prioritize seeking God's kingdom above all else and to be willing to make whatever sacrifices are necessary to enter into its fullness. It also emphasizes the joy and fulfillment that come from knowing and belonging to God's kingdom. Ultimately, the parable encourages us to pursue the kingdom of God with unwavering devotion, trusting in its surpassing value and eternal significance.

99. The Parable of the Workers in the Vineyard

Matthew 20:1-16

Jesus told a parable to His disciples:

"There was a landowner who went out early in the morning to hire workers for his vineyard. He agreed to pay them a denarius for the day's work and sent them into his vineyard.

About nine in the morning, he went out and saw others standing in the marketplace doing nothing. He told them, 'You also go and work in my vineyard, and I will pay you whatever is right.' So they went.

He went out again about noon and at three in the afternoon and did the same thing. About five in the afternoon, he went out and found still others standing around. He asked them, 'Why have you been standing here all day long doing nothing?'

'Because no one has hired us,' they answered.

He said to them, 'You also go and work in my vineyard.'

When evening came, the owner of the vineyard said to his foreman, 'Call the workers and pay them their wages, beginning with the last ones hired and going on to the first.'

The workers who were hired last came and received a denarius, and those who were hired first also received a denarius. When they received it, they began to grumble against the landowner. 'These who were hired last worked only one hour,' they said, 'and you have made them equal to us who have borne the burden of the work and the heat of the day.'

The landowner replied, 'I am not being unfair to you, friend. Didn't you agree to work for a denarius? Take your pay and go. I want to give the one who was hired last the same as I gave you. Don't I have the right to do what I want with my own money? Or are you envious because I am generous?'"

In this parable, Jesus illustrates the generosity and grace of God's kingdom. The landowner's actions challenge the workers' expectations of fairness and highlight God's boundless love and mercy. Just as the landowner's payment was not based on merit but on his own generosity, God's grace is freely given to all who respond to His call, regardless of their past or present circumstances.

100. The Parable of the Vine and the Branches

John 15:1-8

Jesus shared a parable with his disciples:

"I am the true vine, and my Father is the gardener. He cuts off every branch in me that bears no fruit, while every branch that does bear fruit he prunes so that it will be even more fruitful. You are already clean because of the word I have spoken to you. Remain in me, as I also remain in you. No branch can bear fruit by itself; it must remain in the vine. Neither can you bear fruit unless you remain in me.

"I am the vine; you are the branches. If you remain in me and I in you, you will bear much fruit; apart from me, you can do nothing. If you do not remain in me, you are like a branch that is thrown away and withers; such branches are picked up, thrown into the fire and burned. If you remain in me and my words remain in you, ask whatever you wish, and it will be done for you. This is to my Father's glory, that you bear much fruit, showing yourselves to be my disciples."

In this parable, Jesus uses the metaphor of a vine and its branches to illustrate the relationship between Him and His followers. He emphasizes the importance of remaining connected to Him, just as branches are connected to the vine, in order to bear fruit. Jesus is the source of life and sustenance for His disciples, and only by abiding in Him can they experience true spiritual vitality and productivity.

The imagery of pruning highlights the process of spiritual growth and refinement. God, the gardener, removes what is unnecessary or detrimental from the lives of believers so that they can become more fruitful. This parable underscores the vital importance of abiding in Christ and living in communion with Him, which leads to a life characterized by spiritual abundance and effectiveness.

101. The Parable of the Growing Seed

Mark 4:26-29

Jesus told a parable to the crowd:

"The kingdom of God is like a man who scatters seed on the ground. Night and day, whether he sleeps or gets up, the seed sprouts and grows, though he does not know how. All by itself the soil produces grain—first the stalk, then the head, then the full kernel in the head. As soon as the grain is ripe, he puts the sickle to it, because the harvest has come."

In this parable, Jesus compares the kingdom of God to a seed that is sown in the ground. Just as a farmer scatters seed and it grows into a crop without his understanding of the process, the kingdom of God grows and develops mysteriously and gradually.

The farmer's role in the growth of the seed is limited to sowing it in the ground. After that, the growth process is beyond his control and understanding. Similarly, the expansion of God's kingdom is ultimately the work of God Himself, and humans play a role in sowing the seed of the gospel message, but the actual growth and fruition of the kingdom are orchestrated by God's sovereignty.

This parable teaches us about the nature of the kingdom of God and the mysterious way in which it advances. It encourages believers to faithfully sow the seed of the gospel and trust in God's power to bring about spiritual growth and transformation in the hearts of people. Just as the farmer patiently waits for the harvest, we are called to patiently await the fulfillment of God's kingdom purposes, knowing that He is at work in ways we may not fully comprehend.

The End

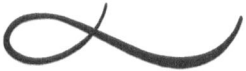